This book is to be returned on or before
the last date stamped below.

Table 2

Antidysrhythmic Drug Dosages

Drug	Mg/Kg PO		Mg/Kg IV	
Atropine	—		0.01–0.03	
Digoxin: Total digitalizing dose†	0.06		0.04	
maintenance§	0.0075–0.01	q12h	0.004–0.006	q12h
Disopyramide	2.0	q12h	—	
Lidocaine	—		1.0	bolus, then 1 mg/Kg/ hr drip
Phenytoin	2.5–5.0	q12h	10.0–15.0*	
Procainamide	—		10.0–15.0*	
Propranolol	0.5–1.5	q6h	0.01–0.1**	
Quinidine Sulfate	7.5–10.0	q6h	—	

  *Give over 1 hour in five divided bolus doses. Watch for hypotension.

  **Give only if electrode catheter is in the heart for emergency pacing.

  †Maximum total digitalizing dose = 1.0 mg.

  §Maximum maintenance dose = 0.125 mg bid.

A Guide to
Cardiac Dysrhythmias in Children

CLINICAL CARDIOLOGY MONOGRAPHS

SERIES CONSULTANTS: J. Willis Hurst, M.D., and Dean T. Mason, M.D.

Cardiac Pacing, Second Edition, edited by Philip Samet and Nabil El-Sherif

The Aorta, edited by Joseph Lindsay, Jr., and J. Willis Hurst

Cardiac Anesthesia, edited by Joel A. Kaplan

Advances in Heart Disease, Volume 2, edited by Dean T. Mason

Atherosclerosis: Its Pediatric Aspects, edited by William B. Strong

Infective Endocarditis, edited by Shahbudin H. Rahimtoola

Hyperlipidemia: Diagnosis and Therapy, edited by Basil M. Rifkind and Robert I. Levy

Cardiac Arrhythmias: Electrophysiologic Basis for Clinical Interpretation, by Yoshio Watanabe and Leonard S. Dreifus

Advances in Heart Disease, Volume 1, edited by Dean T. Mason

Echocardiography: A Teaching Atlas, by Joel M. Felner and Robert C. Schlant

Advances in Electrocardiography, Volume 2, edited by Robert C. Schlant and J. Willis Hurst

Clinical Cardiovascular Physiology, edited by Herbert J. Levine

The Acute Coronary Attack, by J. F. Pantridge, A. A. J. Adgey, J. S. Geddes, and S. W. Webb

The Peripheral Circulations, edited by Robert Zelis

Rheumatic Fever and Streptococcal Infection, by Gene H. Stollerman

Shock in Myocardial Infarction, edited by Rolf M. Gunnar, Henry S. Loeb, and Shahbudin H. Rahimtoola

Noninvasive Cardiology, edited by Arnold M. Weissler

Advances in Cardiovascular Surgery, edited by John W. Kirklin

Myocardial Disease, edited by Noble O. Fowler

Advances in Electrocardiography, Volume 1, edited by Robert C. Schlant and J. Willis Hurst

A Guide to
Cardiac Dysrhythmias in Children

Arthur Garson, Jr., M.D.
Assistant Professor of Pediatrics

Paul C. Gillette, M.D.
Assistant Professor of Pediatrics

Dan G. McNamara, M.D.
Professor of Pediatrics

The Lillie Frank Abercrombie Section of Pediatric Cardiology
Baylor College of Medicine and Texas Children's Hospital
Houston, Texas

GRUNE & STRATTON
A Subsidiary of Harcourt Brace Jovanovich, Publishers
New York   London   Toronto   Sydney   San Francisco

This work was made possible by a grant from
The J. S. Abercrombie Foundation.

Grune & Stratton, Inc.
111 Fifth Avenue
New York, New York 10003

Distributed in the United Kingdom by
Academic Press, Inc. (London) Ltd.
24/28 Oval Road, London NW 1

Library of Congress Catalog Number 80-16937
International Standard Book Number 0-8089-1261-5
Printed in the United States of America

Contents

PREFACE

This guide contains the most common disturbances of heart rate, rhythm, and impulse conduction in children. It is intended to serve as a quick reference to specific dysrhythmias rather than as a complete textbook of pediatric electrocardiography.

The book begins with an outline for the systematic interpretation of cardiac dysrhythmias in children. In addition to providing a method for approaching the electrocardiogram, this section is intended to be the starting point for practical use of the book. The reader is urged to read this section first. With the use of information provided in this section, a differential diagnosis of a dysrhythmia can be formulated and then the reader can refer to the Contents to find the specific dysrhythmias in the differential diagnosis. In this section only, drawings of electrocardiograms were made to facilitate comparison.

After examples of sinus rhythm, the book is divided into three sections: disturbances in cardiac rate and rhythm, disturbances in cardiac conduction, and artificial pacemakers. Table 1 provides normal values for electrocardiographic findings in children, and Table 2 lists current recommendations for acute and chronic antidysrhythmic drug dosages. These tables, as well as the outlines of dysrhythmias with a regular R–R interval and dysrhythmias with an irregular R–R interval are reproduced on pocket cards.

The subsection on each dysrhythmia begins with a description of the surface electrocardiographic criteria for diagnosis, the common clinical situations in which the dysrhythmia may be found, a differential diagnosis, and suggested management. Sample electrocardiographic tracings taken from actual patients are recorded at usual paper speed (25 mm/sec) with usual standardization (1 mv = 10 mm). In the legend for each tracing is a short history of the patient and an interpretation which indicates the specific findings.

We would like to dedicate this book to Mr. Americo Simonelli, Senior Technician, Electrocardiographic Laboratory, Texas Children's Hospital. His standards of excellence in the recording of electrocardiograms from children of all ages are demonstrated throughout these pages. Our assistant and advisor, Ms. Harriett Self, has worked tirelessly on the preparation of the manuscript. To her goes a special expression of our gratitude.

Systematic Interpretation of Cardiac Dysrhythmias in Children

Deciphering a child's dysrhythmia can be both a challenging and rewarding experience. If a systematic approach is used in interpretation, an electrocardiogram that at first glance seems bizarre may actually be relatively simple. Certain principles are helpful in the analysis of the cardiac rhythm in children. We have developed a step-by-step method of diagnosis which, while not including every possible dysrhythmia, will place most rhythm disturbances in a single category. In analyzing the ECG, certain questions must be answered sequentially (Fig. 1).

This method differs from most others in that it begins with the QRS complex. The QRS is the most obvious feature of the ECG and, in actual practice, the first determination made is usually the regularity of the QRS complexes. We have used hand-drawn ECG tracings in the teaching of this method. These tracings have several advantages. First, they allow us to vary one part of the ECG at a time while keeping all other parts constant; for example, keeping the QRS rate and P rate exactly the same while varying only the P axis. Therefore, focus is directed at the important teaching point rather than at the unimportant slight change in rate or QRS morphology. The second advantage is that the tracings are easy to read, without wandering baselines or electrical interference.

The use of this method requires no expertise with the electrophysiologic principles that underlie the ECG. This is a stepwise deductive method used by pediatric cardiologists. It can be learned by anyone who knows the basics of the ECG in adults or children: morphology, rate, axis, and duration of both the P wave and QRS complex. Once learned, it is a method which may be easily and quickly reviewed by clinicians who encounter dysrhythmias infrequently in children. When the questions in Figure 1 are answered, the dysrhythmias will be identified.

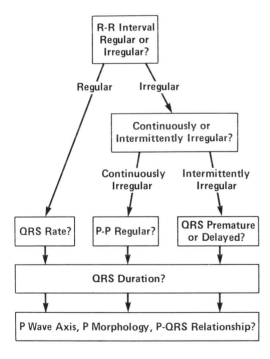

Figure 1.
Schema for Interpretation of Dysrhythmias

REGULAR vs. IRREGULAR RHYTHM

The first step is to decide if the ventricular rate (R-R interval) is regular. We consider a rhythm to be regular if the R-R intervals in the ECG vary by less than 0.08 seconds (see Fig. 2). The examples shown in the figures are idealized drawings taken from the ECGs of different 4-year-old patients. For patients in the 4 to 5-year age range, the normal QRS rate ranges from 60 to 150/min, the normal PR interval is 0.11 to 0.15 sec, and the normal QRS duration is 0.05 to 0.09 sec.

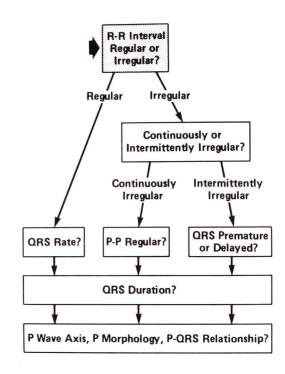

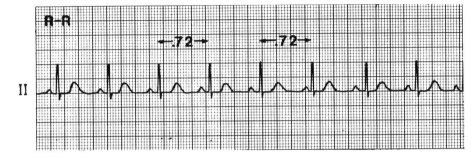

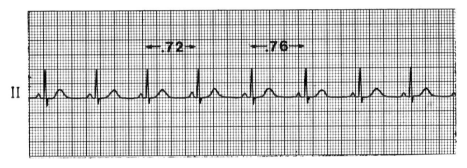

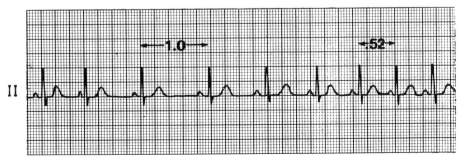

Figure 2.

Top tracing: Sinus rhythm; absolutely regular R-R interval of 0.72 sec (QRS rate = 85/min).

Middle tracing: Sinus rhythm; first three R-R intervals are 0.72 sec, followed by three R-R intervals of 0.76 sec. Since the R-R intervals vary by 0.08 sec or less, this is considered to be a regular rhythm.

Bottom tracing: Sinus arrhythmia; the R-R intervals vary from 0.52 to 1.0 sec. This is a markedly irregular rhythm.

5

VARIATION IN QRS RATE

If the ventricular rate is regular, the answers to three further questions will categorize the rhythm. The first question is whether the ventricular rate is decreased, normal, or increased for a child of the patient's age. For example, in Figure 3 three sample ECGs are shown, each taken from a 4-year-old patient. The ventricular rates are 50/min, 85/min, and 180/min. For a 4-year-old child a ventricular rate of 50/min is bradycardia and 180/min is tachycardia.

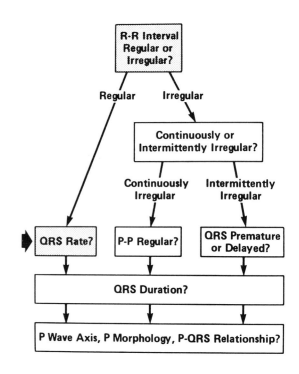

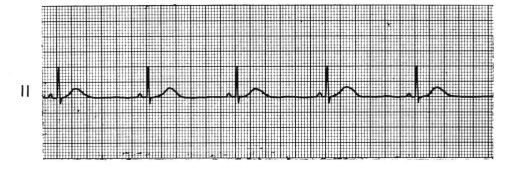

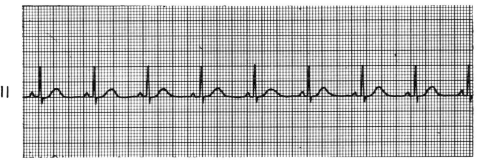

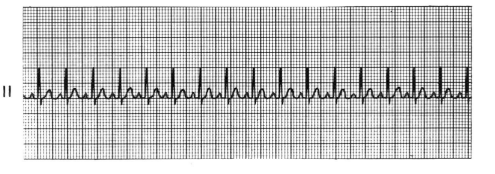

Figure 3.

Top tracing: Sinus bradycardia; QRS rate is 50/min.

Middle tracing: Sinus rhythm; QRS rate is 85/min.

Bottom tracing: Sinus tachycardia; QRS rate is 180/min.

The second question to be answered is whether the QRS duration is normal or prolonged. If the QRS duration is prolonged, the specific morphology must be determined. In a 4-year-old, the upper limit of normal for QRS duration is 0.09 sec. Any QRS complex that is longer than 0.09 sec is prolonged. An abnormally long QRS complex may have one of four distinct morphologies (Figs. 4 and 5). It is helpful to distinguish among these different morphologies by looking at leads V_1 and V_6. In complete right bundle branch block (CRBBB), the initial 0.04 sec shows a rapid, normal deflection and the terminal forces are inscribed slowly (wide QRS). These terminal forces are directed anteriorly and to the right (positive in V_1 and negative in V_6) because the right ventricle has delayed activation. Therefore in CRBBB, in V_1 the complex is mainly positive with an rSR′ morphology. In complete left bundle branch block (CLBBB), the delayed terminal forces are directed posteriorly and to the left because the left ventricle has delayed activation; thus in V_1 the complex is mainly negative, and in V_6 it is mainly positive with an R-R′ morphology (Fig. 4).

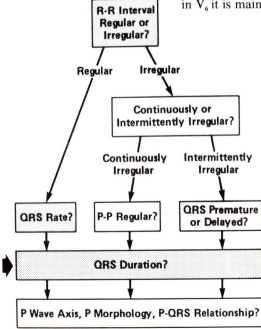

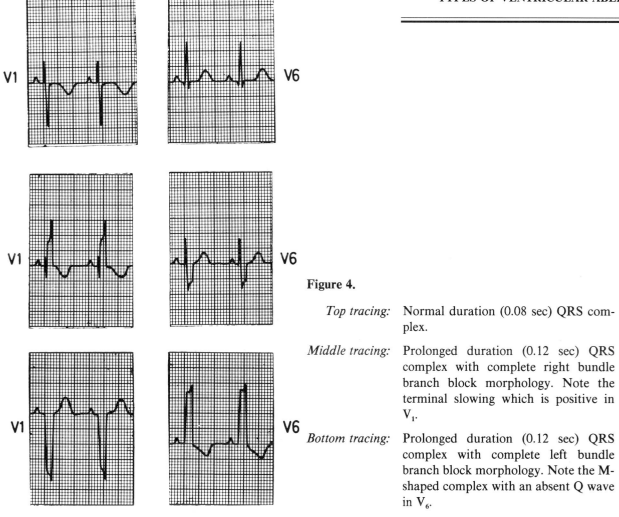

Figure 4.

Top tracing: Normal duration (0.08 sec) QRS complex.

Middle tracing: Prolonged duration (0.12 sec) QRS complex with complete right bundle branch block morphology. Note the terminal slowing which is positive in V_1.

Bottom tracing: Prolonged duration (0.12 sec) QRS complex with complete left bundle branch block morphology. Note the M-shaped complex with an absent Q wave in V_6.

TYPES OF VENTRICULAR ABERRATION

In the Wolff-Parkinson-White syndrome, the PR interval is short and the abnormally prolonged QRS complex is inscribed slowly in the initial 0.02 to 0.04 sec. This slow initial deflection is called the "delta" wave. The remainder of the QRS complex is inscribed rapidly and normally.

The QRS complex of diffuse intraventricular conduction delay found in quinidine toxicity, myocarditis, hypoglycemia, myocardial ischemia, and hyperkalemia involves delay in all phases of depolarization and the inscription of the entire QRS complex is prolonged (Fig. 5).

Figure 5.

Top tracing: Prolonged duration (0.12 sec) QRS complex with Wolff-Parkinson-White morphology. The PR interval is short (0.08 sec). The initial 0.04 sec of the QRS has a slurred upstroke—the "delta" wave. The latter part of the QRS is normal.

Bottom tracing: Prolonged duration (0.12 sec) QRS complex with morphology of diffuse intraventricular conduction delay. This is a wide QRS complex without the specific morphology of CRBBB, CLBBB, or Wolff-Parkinson-White.

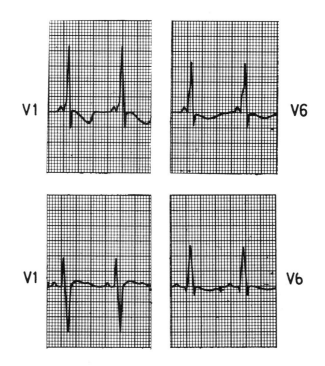

The third question to be answered concerns atrial activity. When the atria depolarize, one of three patterns is observed in the ECG (Fig. 6):

1. P waves—distinct depolarizations, normally 0.03 to 0.08 sec in duration and more pointed than T waves.
2. Flutter waves—0.09 to 0.18 sec in duration and occurring in succession, giving the impression of a "sawtooth" baseline. Flutter waves may not be visible in all ECG leads; the most likely leads to show flutter waves are II, III, aV_F, and V_1.
3. Fibrillation—coarse or fine irregular oscillations of the baseline without other demonstrable atrial activity.

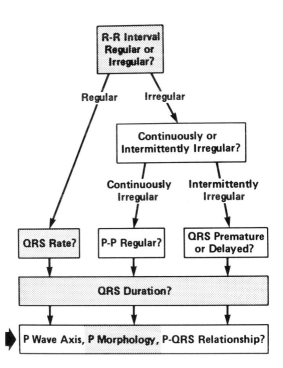

MORPHOLOGY OF ATRIAL DEPOLARIZATION

III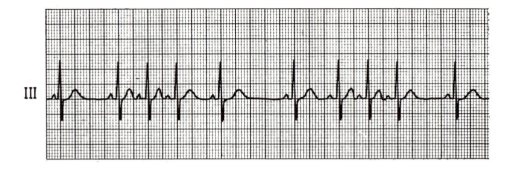

III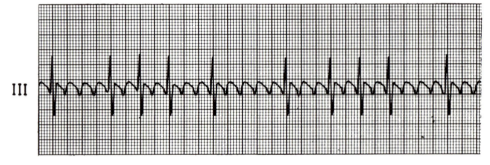

III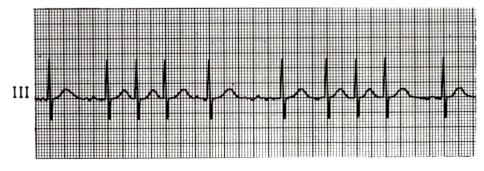

Top tracing: Sinus arrhythmia; a P wave precedes each QRS complex.

Middle tracing: Atrial flutter with varying type II second degree AV block; flutter waves are visible throughout the tracing

Bottom tracing: Atrial fibrillation; note the fine oscillations in the baseline.

Figure 6.

If P waves are visible, the P wave axis must be determined. With the P wave, it is only necessary to determine the quadrant of the axis (Figs. 7 and 8). If the patient has atrial situs solitus and the axis is 0° to 90°, the impulse arises high in the right atrium and this represents sinus rhythm. If the axis is 91° to 180°, the impulse originates high in the left atrium; 180° to 269°, low in the left atrium (Fig. 7); and 270° to 359°, low in the right atrium (Fig. 8). In junctional or ventricular dysrhythmias with intact retrograde conduction through the bundle of His and atrioventricular (AV) node, the "retrograde" P wave originates atrial depolarization from the region of the AV node and has an axis of 270° to 359° (Fig. 8). If the patient has atrial situs inversus and normal sinus rhythm, the P wave axis is 91° to 180°. If the right and left arm leads are reversed on the patient with sinus rhythm and situs solitus, the P wave axis is also 91° to 180°.

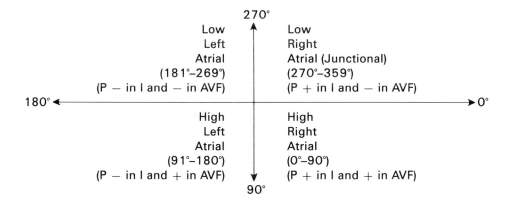

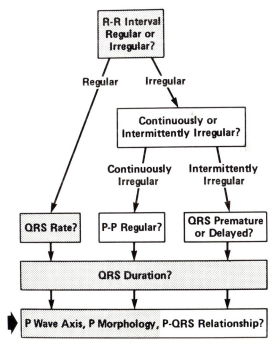

Figure 7.

===
P WAVE AXIS
===

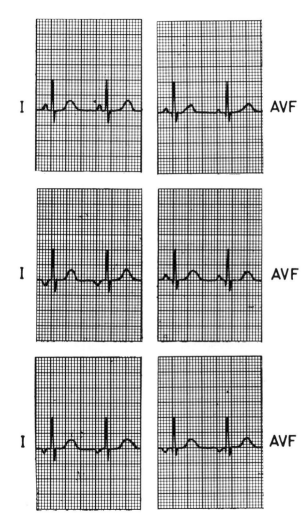

Top tracing: Sinus rhythm; P wave axis 0°–90°.

Middle tracing: High left atrial rhythm; P wave axis 91°–180°.

Bottom tracing: Low left atrial rhythm; P wave axis 181°–269°.

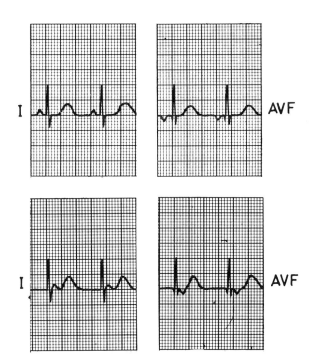

I   AVF

I   AVF

Figure 8.

Top tracing: Low right atrial rhythm; P wave axis 270°–359°.

Bottom tracing: Junctional rhythm; P wave axis 270°–359° with P wave following QRS complex.

P-QRS RELATIONSHIP

Finally, the relationship of the atrial depolarizations to the QRS complexes must be determined. Either the atrial depolarizations are related in a regular way to the QRS complexes, or the atrial depolarizations are unrelated to the QRS complexes (AV dissociation). If an atrial depolarization precedes each QRS complex with a PR interval of 0.30 sec or less, we assume that the atrial depolarization conducted through the His bundle and caused the ventricular depolarization (Fig. 9). If an atrial depolarization follows each QRS complex with a constant R-P interval of 0.30 sec or less (and an axis of 270° to 359°), we assume that the AV junction or ventricle initiated the depolarization and the impulse conducted retrogradely through the AV node and depolarized the atrium. One other type of P-QRS relationship occurs if there are more P waves than QRS complexes: if the R-R interval is regular and the P-P interval (atrial rate) is a constant multiple of the ventricular rate (every second, third, or fourth atrial depolarization is followed by a QRS complex), the diagnosis is second degree AV block. In this case, each ventricular depolarization is caused by an atrial depolarization.

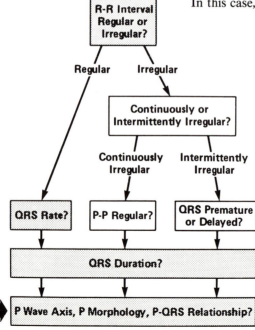

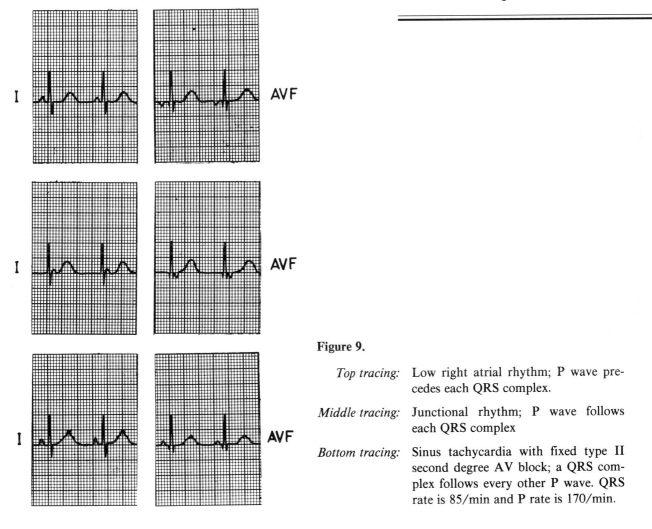

Figure 9.

Top tracing: Low right atrial rhythm; P wave precedes each QRS complex.

Middle tracing: Junctional rhythm; P wave follows each QRS complex

Bottom tracing: Sinus tachycardia with fixed type II second degree AV block; a QRS complex follows every other P wave. QRS rate is 85/min and P rate is 170/min.

AV DISSOCIATION

If the atrial and ventricular depolarizations are unrelated, the diagnosis is AV dissociation. AV dissociation occurs in several dysrhythmias of entirely different mechanisms. Therefore, AV dissociation should never be the only diagnosis in the interpretation of an ECG. There are three major causes for AV dissociation (Figs. 10 and 11):

1. Slowing of sinus or atrial rhythm with junctional rhythm occuring at a normal junctional rate. If retrograde conduction to the atria does not occur during junctional rhythm, AV dissociation may occur, with the slow sinus beats continuing to depolarize the atria while the impulses arising in the junction depolarize the ventricles. (Fig. 10)
2. An accelerated junctional or a ventricular rhythm without retrograde conduction results in an abnormally rapid ventricular rate with a normal sinus rate. (Fig. 10)
3. Complete AV block is the best example of AV dissociation because, by definition, the atria and ventricles are unrelated. (Fig. 11)

It is possible to have the atria and ventricles beating at exactly the same rate and a constant PR interval with no conduction from atria to ventricles. This is called "isorhythmic" or "isochronic" dissociation. (Fig. 11) The only way to prove the existence of isochronic dissociation is to find, in a long rhythm strip, that one of the two rates changes (atria or ventricles) and the other stays the same. For example, if the P-P interval lengthens and the R-R interval remains constant, AV dissociation will become evident.

Figure 10.

Top tracing: Sinus rhythm followed by junctional rhythm with AV dissociation; the first three complexes are sinus rhythm at a rate of 85/min. The sinus rate then slows to 55/min (P-P interval = 1.09 sec). The patient's normal junctional rate of 60/min (R-R interval = 0.72 sec) is usually suppressed by the faster sinus rate. At this time, however, the junctional rate is faster than the sinus rate and the junction assumes the function of the pacemaker. The sinus P waves continue dissociated through the tracing because in this patient there is no retrograde conduction to the atrium from the junction, so sinus rhythm is not disturbed.

Bottom tracing: Sinus rhythm followed by accelerated junctional rhythm with AV dissociation. The first three complexes are sinus rhythm at a rate of 85/min. The sinus rate remains 85/min (sinus P waves marked by arrows every 0.72 sec), but the AV junction develops an abnormally rapid rate of 100/min (R-R interval 0.60 sec) and assumes the pacemaker function. The P waves and QRS complexes are dissociated because there is no retrograde conduction from the junction to the atria; however, conduction is intact from atria to ventri-

cles. A short R-R interval (0.48 sec) is found when a sinus P wave occurs a sufficient time after the preceding QRS complex so that the AV node is not refractory and AV conduction can occur. This is a sinus "capture" beat; accelerated junctional rhythm resumes after the capture beat.

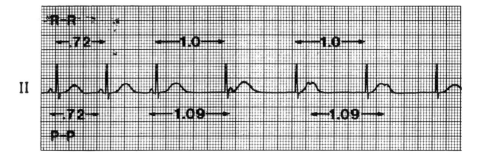

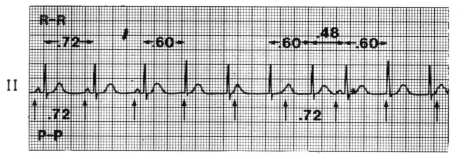

Top tracing: Complete AV block; junctional rate is 60/min (R-R interval 1.0 sec); the atrial rate is 85/min (P-P interval 0.72 sec), and the P waves and QRS complexes are dissociated because there is no conduction through the AV node in either antegrade or retrograde direction. If antegrade conduction was intact, two P waves (arrows) should have changed the R-R interval (see Fig. 10, bottom). The R-R interval was not influenced by the intevening P waves and therefore the P waves probably did not conduct to the ventricles.

Bottom tracing: Complete AV block with isochronic dissociation; the R-R intervals remain absolutely constant at 0.72 sec and the P-P intervals begin at 0.72 sec. However, the P-P intervals lengthen to 0.76 sec with a shortening PR interval and the R-R interval is unaffected. The change in atrial rate without a corresponding change in ventricular rate is the clue that the first three P waves most likely were not conducted to the ventricles but only appeared to be because the atria and ventricles were beating independently at exactly the same rate ("isochronic" dissociation).

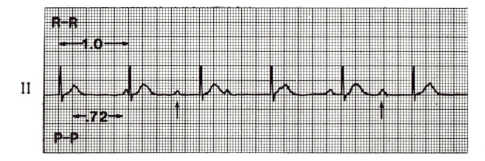

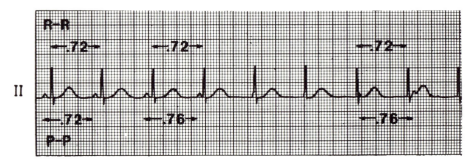

Figure 11.

If the R-R intervals are irregular, they can either be irregular continuously or there can be a basic, regular R-R interval into which an irregular R-R interval is intermittently introduced (Fig. 12).

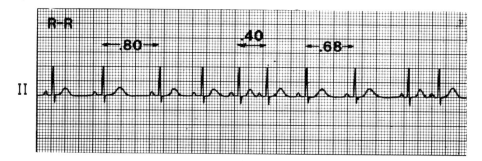

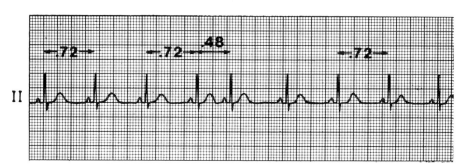

Figure 12.

Top tracing: Sinus arrhythmia; the R-R intervals vary throughout the tracing. This is "continuously irregular."

Bottom tracing: Sinus rhythm with premature atrial contraction; the R-R intervals are basically constant but are interrupted by an irregular R-R interval. This is "intermittently irregular."

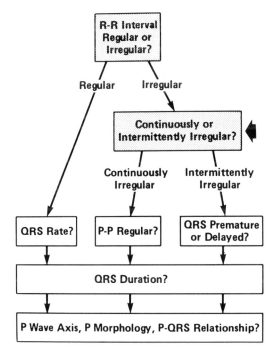

CONTINUOUSLY IRREGULAR RHYTHMS

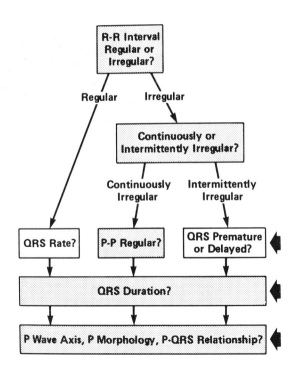

If the R-R interval varies continuously, the next question to be answered is whether the P-P intervals are regular. Next the QRS duration should be ascertained and, if the QRS is continuously irregular, the P wave axis, P morphology, and P-QRS relationship should be determined (Fig. 13). In pediatrics, if the P-P intervals vary, generally the atrial and ventricular depolarizations are related and therefore the R-R interval also will vary. The two most common causes of irregular P-P and R-R intervals are sinus arrhythmia and wandering pacemaker. In sinus arrhythmia, the P wave axis varies between 0° and 90°. In wandering pacemaker, P waves are not always present; when P waves are present, the P wave axis may vary throughout the four quadrants. Of course, atrial fibrillation is the well known "irregularly irregular" rhythm and falls into the category of irregular R-R intervals.

If the R-R interval is irregular but the P-P interval is regular, the most likely diagnosis is second degree AV block of a type in which the R-R intervals vary. In typical type I second degree AV block (Wenckebach), the PR intervals progressively lengthen and the R-R intervals progressively shorten until an atrial depolarization occurs without a following QRS complex, and then the cycle begins again. In type II second degree AV block, the PR intervals remain constant but the R-R intervals may vary if the number of atrial depolarizations that are conducted to the ventricles vary (Fig. 13). Each type of AV block can occur with any type of supraventricular rhythm—either sinus or ectopic atrial rhythm, supraventricular tachycardia, or atrial flutter.

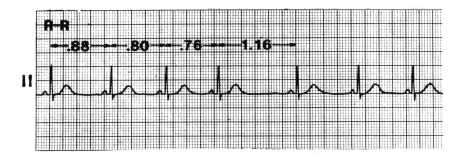

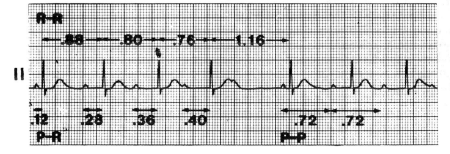

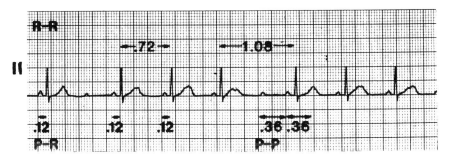

Figure 13.

Top tracing: Sinus arrhythmia; R-R intervals vary from 0.76 to 1.16 sec and each QRS complex is preceded by a P wave with a constant PR interval.

Middle tracing: Sinus rhythm with type I second degree AV block (Wenckebach); the R-R intervals are identical to those in the top tracing and the PR interval lengthens until a P wave is not followed by a QRS (arrow).

Bottom tracing: Sinus tachycardia with varying type II second degree AV block; the atrial rate is 167 (P-P interval = 0.36 sec), and the R-R interval varies from 0.90 with 2 : 1 block to 1.08 with 4 : 1 block.

INTERMITTENTLY IRREGULAR: PREMATURE vs. DELAYED QRS

If there is a basic, regular R-R interval that is interrupted intermittently, the initial question to be answered is whether the first irregular R-R interval is shorter or longer than the basic, regular R-R interval (Fig. 14). In order to be considered irregular, the R-R interval must vary from the basic R-R interval by 0.04 sec or more.

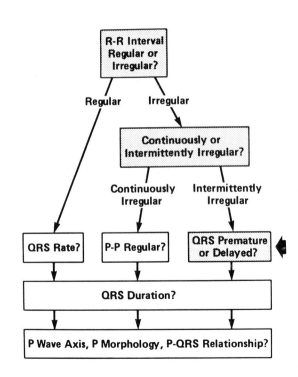

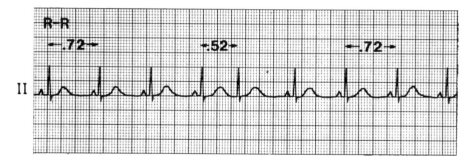

Figure 14.

Top tracing: Sinus rhythm with premature junctional contraction; basic R-R interval is regular at 0.72 sec and is interrupted by a premature QRS with an R-R interval of 0.52 sec.

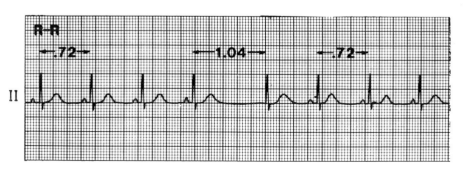

Bottom tracing: Sinus rhythm with sinus pause and junctional escape beat; basic R-R interval is regular at 0.72 sec and is interrupted by a delayed QRS with an R-R interval of 1.04 sec.

INTERMITTENTLY IRREGULAR: PREMATURE QRS

If the QRS is premature by at least 0.04 sec, the R-R interval that follows the premature QRS may be prolonged. The degree of prolongation has been used to distinguish among types of premature beat. In children, any type of premature beat may be followed by a "compensatory pause" and so the degree of prolongation is of little value.

The QRS duration is determined next. If the QRS duration is normal, the premature QRS can have one of three causes:

1. Intermittent conduction of a sinus beat. In the presence of atrial or junctional rhythm, the sinus node continues to depolarize. If the early QRS is preceded by a P wave with a normal axis (0° to 90°) and the PR interval is 0.30 sec or less, the sinus node depolarization has conducted to the atria, causing the P wave, and the atrial impulse has conducted to the ventricles (so-called "sinus capture").

2. In either sinus, atrial, or junctional rhythm, if the early QRS is preceded by a premature P wave and a PR interval of 0.30 sec or less, this is a premature atrial contraction.

3. If the QRS is not preceded by a P wave, this is a premature junctional contraction (Fig. 15).

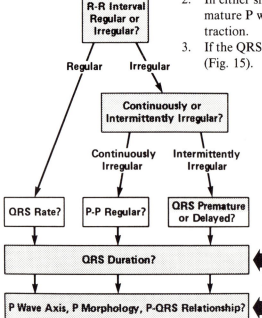

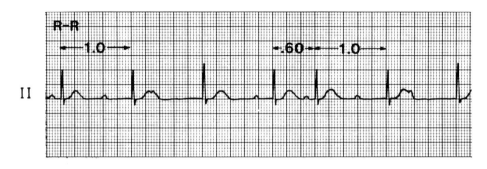

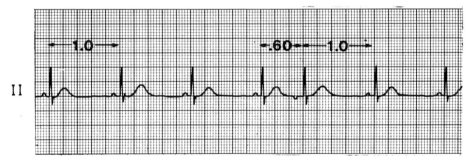

Figure 15.

Top tracing: Sinus rhythm with advanced second degree AV block and junctional escape rhythm; the basic R-R interval is 1.0 sec (junctional rhythm at 60/min). The premature QRS is due to a sinus "capture" beat (see Fig. 11). This is the only P wave that conducts. All of the other P waves are blocked.

Middle tracing: Sinus rhythm with premature atrial contraction; the basic R-R interval is 1.0 sec (sinus rhythm at 60/min). The premature QRS is preceded by a P wave which is negative in lead II; this is a premature atrial contraction originating from an inferior location in the atria.

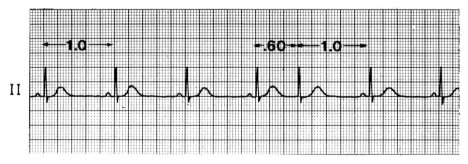

Bottom tracing: Sinus rhythm with premature junctional contraction; the basic R-R interval is 1.0 sec (sinus rhythm at 60/min). The premature QRS is not preceded by a P wave.

INTERMITTENTLY IRREGULAR: PREMATURE QRS

If the premature QRS has a prolonged duration, there are three possible causes which are similar to those for a normal duration QRS:

1. Sinus capture with aberration
2. Premature atrial contraction with aberration
3. Premature ventricular contraction

It is possible to have a premature QRS complex without a preceding P wave due to a premature junctional contraction with aberration. It is impossible, however, on the surface ECG in children to distinguish a premature junctional contraction with aberration from a premature ventricular contraction (Fig. 16). Therefore, we have chosen to classify all QRS complexes that are premature and have a prolonged duration without preceding P waves as premature ventricular contractions.

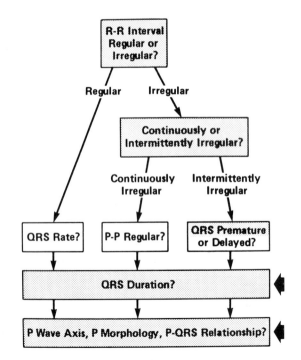

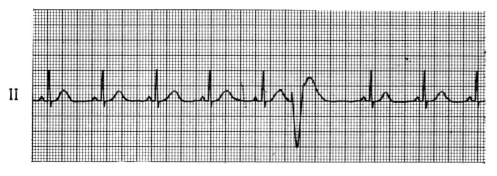

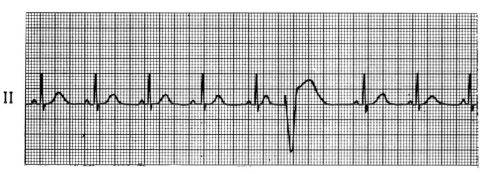

Figure 16.

Top tracing: Sinus rhythm and premature ventricular contraction; basic R-R interval interrupted by a premature QRS with prolonged duration.

Bottom tracing: Sinus rhythm and premature junctional contraction with aberration; basic R-R interval interrupted by a premature QRS with prolonged duration. These two dysrhythmias are indistinguishable on the surface ECG.

INTERMITTENTLY IRREGULAR: DELAYED QRS

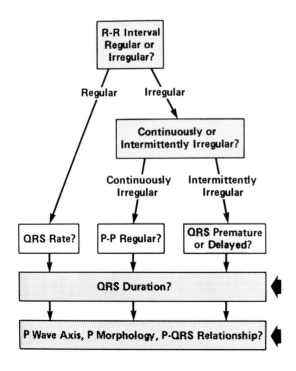

R-R Interval
Regular or
Irregular?

Regular   Irregular

Continuously or
Intermittently Irregular?

Continuously   Intermittently
Irregular   Irregular

QRS Rate?   P-P Regular?   QRS Premature or Delayed?

QRS Duration?

P Wave Axis, P Morphology, P-QRS Relationship?

If the QRS is not premature but rather delayed by 0.04 sec or more, the QRS duration should be determined. If the QRS duration is normal, the answers to three questions will classify the rhythm. The first question refers to the basic supraventricular rhythm: (a) in second degree AV block, the supraventricular rhythm continues uninterrupted; (b) in a nonconducted premature atrial contraction, a different morphology P wave is introduced prematurely; and (c) with a "pause" in the supraventricular rhythm, no atrial activity is observed (Figs. 17 and 18).

Second, what is the R-R interval from the delayed QRS complex back to the immediately preceding QRS? In type II second degree AV block, the R-R interval is twice the basic R-R interval; in a nonconducted premature atrial contraction, the R-R interval is less than twice the basic R-R interval. While most premature atrial contractions can be followed by either a compensatory or a noncompensatory pause, virtually all nonconducted premature atrial contractions have less than a fully compensatory pause. Therefore, both the P-P and R-R intervals should be less than twice the basic R-R interval. In a "pause," the R-R interval can be of any duration but is always longer than the basic R-R interval (Fig. 17).

The third question concerns the atrial activity immediately preceding the delayed QRS complex. In AV block, the delayed QRS is preceded by a supraventricular P wave which is identical to that seen in the basic rhythm. In a nonconducted premature atrial contraction, the delayed QRS is also preceded by a supraventricular P wave which is identical to that seen in the basic supraventricular rhythm. In a pause with atrial escape, the delayed QRS is preceded by a P wave with a different axis and morphology from the basic P wave. In a pause with junctional escape, the delayed QRS is not preceded by a P wave.

If the QRS complex is delayed and the QRS duration is prolonged, the most common rhythm is a pause with ventricular escape (Fig. 18).

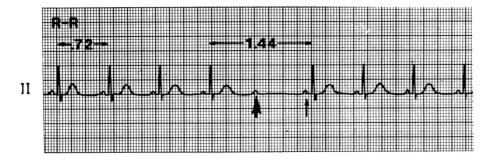

Figure 17.

Top tracing: Sinus rhythm with type II second degree AV block; the basic R-R interval is interrupted by an irregular R-R interval which is exactly twice the basic R-R interval. Sinus rhythm continues after the last regular QRS (large arrow); sinus rhythm initiates the QRS, which is delayed (small arrow).

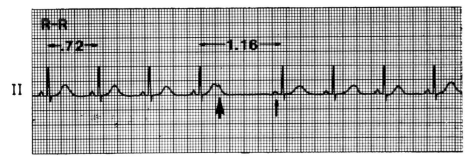

Middle tracing: Sinus rhythm with nonconducted premature atrial contraction; the basic R-R interval is interrupted by an irregular R-R interval which is less than twice the basic R-R interval. The last regular QRS complex is followed by a premature P wave (large arrow); sinus rhythm initiates the QRS, which is delayed (small arrow).

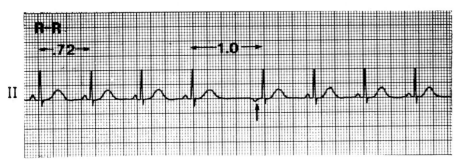

Bottom tracing: Sinus rhythm with sinus pause and low atrial escape beat; the basic R-R interval is interrupted by an irregular R-R interval which is greater than the basic R-R interval. The last regular QRS complex is not followed by a P wave. An inverted P wave (small arrow) precedes the delayed QRS, indicating that this is a low atrial escape beat.

31

Figure 18.

Top tracing: Sinus rhythm with sinus pause and junctional escape beat; the basic R-R interval is interrupted by an irregular R-R interval which is greater than the basic R-R interval and also greater than the R-R interval in low atrial escape (see Fig. 17, bottom). This is because the junctional escape rate is slower than the atrial escape rate; the last regular QRS complex is not followed by a P wave; and no P wave precedes the delayed QRS, indicating that this is a junctional escape beat.

Bottom tracing: Sinus rhythm with sinus pause and ventricular escape beat; the basic R-R interval is interrupted by an irregular R-R interval which is greater than the basic R-R interval and also greater than the R-R interval in either low atrial or junctional escape. The last regular QRS complex is not followed by a P wave. No P wave precedes the delayed QRS, which has prolonged duration, indicating that this is a ventricular escape beat.

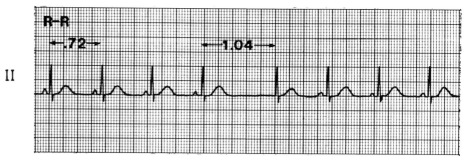

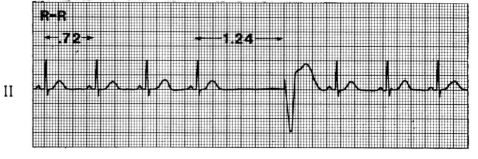

With this background, the major common cardiac rhythm disturbances in children can be better understood. The dysrhythmias are discussed in fourteen categories. Assignment into a category depends upon:

1. Regularity of the R-R interval
2. QRS rate
3. QRS duration

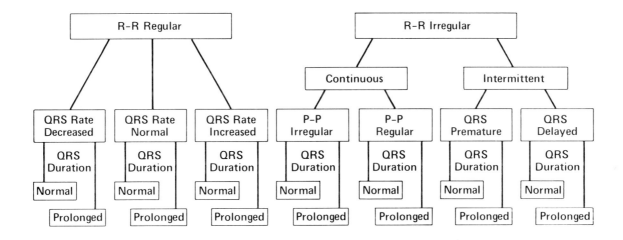

A diagram of the categories is shown below. In the following discussion, dysrhythmia categories are grouped by whether the R-R interval is regular, continuously irregular, or intermittently irregular. Each category is discussed separately with criteria provided for each of the dysrhythmias in the category. Sample hand-drawn ECG tracings are also included with each category to facilitate comparison between dysrhythmias. ECG tracings from actual patients are provided with the expanded discussion of each dysrhythmia at the end of the book.

Figure 19. Dysrhythmias with a Regular R–R Interval

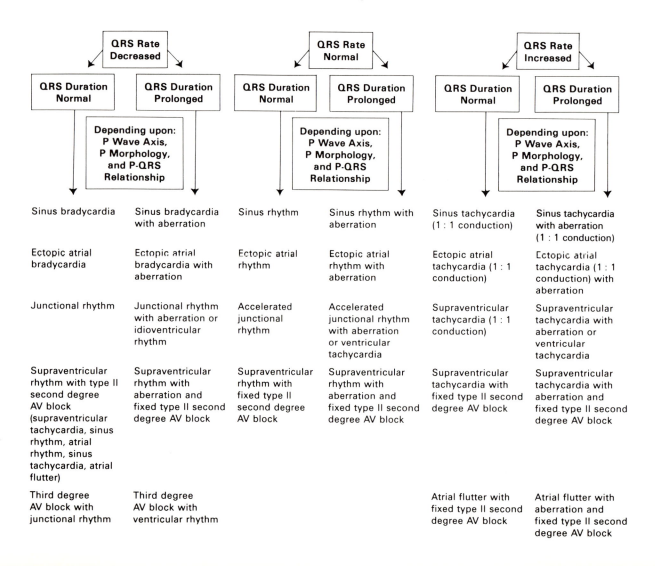

QRS Rate Decreased		QRS Rate Normal		QRS Rate Increased	
QRS Duration Normal	**QRS Duration Prolonged**	**QRS Duration Normal**	**QRS Duration Prolonged**	**QRS Duration Normal**	**QRS Duration Prolonged**
	Depending upon: P Wave Axis, P Morphology, and P-QRS Relationship		Depending upon: P Wave Axis, P Morphology, and P-QRS Relationship		Depending upon: P Wave Axis, P Morphology, and P-QRS Relationship
Sinus bradycardia	Sinus bradycardia with aberration	Sinus rhythm	Sinus rhythm with aberration	Sinus tachycardia (1 : 1 conduction)	Sinus tachycardia with aberration (1 : 1 conduction)
Ectopic atrial bradycardia	Ectopic atrial bradycardia with aberration	Ectopic atrial rhythm	Ectopic atrial rhythm with aberration	Ectopic atrial tachycardia (1 : 1 conduction)	Ectopic atrial tachycardia (1 : 1 conduction) with aberration
Junctional rhythm	Junctional rhythm with aberration or idioventricular rhythm	Accelerated junctional rhythm	Accelerated junctional rhythm with aberration or ventricular tachycardia	Supraventricular tachycardia (1 : 1 conduction)	Supraventricular tachycardia with aberration or ventricular tachycardia
Supraventricular rhythm with type II second degree AV block (supraventricular tachycardia, sinus rhythm, atrial rhythm, sinus tachycardia, atrial flutter)	Supraventricular rhythm with aberration and fixed type II second degree AV block	Supraventricular rhythm with fixed type II second degree AV block	Supraventricular rhythm with aberration and fixed type II second degree AV block	Supraventricular tachycardia with fixed type II second degree AV block	Supraventricular tachycardia with aberration and fixed type II second degree AV block
Third degree AV block with junctional rhythm	Third degree AV block with ventricular rhythm			Atrial flutter with fixed type II second degree AV block	Atrial flutter with aberration and fixed type II second degree AV block

Figure 21. Dysrhythmias with an Intermittently Irregular R–R Interval

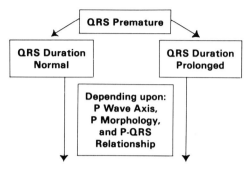

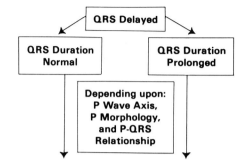

Ectopic atrial or junctional rhythm with sinus capture

Sinus, ectopic atrial, or junctional rhythm with premature atrial contraction

Sinus, ectopic atrial, or junctional rhythm with premature junctional contraction

Ectopic atrial or junctional rhythm with sinus capture and aberration

Sinus, ectopic atrial, or junctional rhythm with premature atrial contraction and aberration

Sinus, ectopic atrial, or junctional rhythm with premature ventricular contraction

Supraventricular rhythm with intermittent type II second degree AV block

Supraventricular rhythm with nonconducted premature atrial contraction

Pause in supraventricular rhythm with ectopic atrial escape

Pause in supraventricular rhythm with junctional escape

Pause in supraventricular rhythm with ventricular escape

Figure 20. Dysrhythmias with a Continuously Irregular R–R Interval

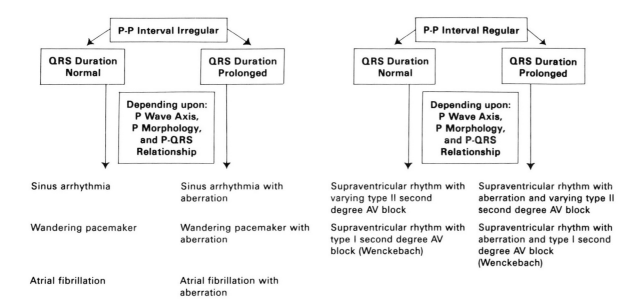

Sinus arrhythmia

Wandering pacemaker

Atrial fibrillation

Sinus arrhythmia with aberration

Wandering pacemaker with aberration

Atrial fibrillation with aberration

Supraventricular rhythm with varying type II second degree AV block

Supraventricular rhythm with type I second degree AV block (Wenckebach)

Supraventricular rhythm with aberration and varying type II second degree AV block

Supraventricular rhythm with aberration and type I second degree AV block (Wenckebach)

R-R INTERVAL   REGULAR
QRS RATE   DECREASED
QRS DURATION   NORMAL

(See Figs. 22–24.)

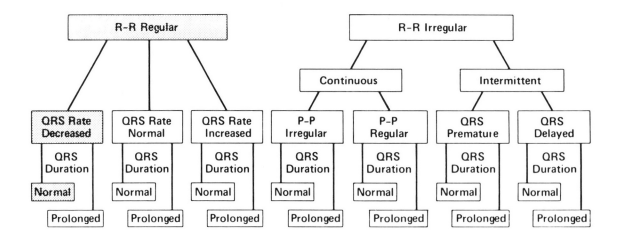

- SINUS BRADYCARDIA

    P wave precedes each QRS complex with normal P wave axis (0° to 90°).

- ECTOPIC ATRIAL BRADYCARDIA

    P wave precedes each QRS complex with abnormal P wave axis (91° to 359°).

- JUNCTIONAL RHYTHM

    Sinus P rate less than QRS rate with AV dissociation, or "retrograde" P wave (axis 270° to 359°) follows some or all QRS complexes with R-P interval <0.30 sec.

- SUPRAVENTRICULAR RHYTHM WITH FIXED TYPE II
  SECOND DEGREE AV BLOCK

    P rate is a multiple of QRS rate with a fixed relationship of P waves to QRS complexes. (Every second, third, or fourth P wave precedes a QRS complex with the same PR interval.) The supraventricular rhythm which is blocked must then be ascertained:

1. *Sinus rhythm with AV block:* P axis and P rate are normal for age.
2. *Atrial rhythm with AV block:* P axis is abnormal and P rate is normal.
3. *Sinus tachycardia with AV block:* P axis is normal and P rate is increased (≤ 230/min).
4. *Supraventricular tachycardia with AV block:* P axis is abnormal and P rate is increased, or P axis is normal and P rate is >230 min.
5. *Atrial flutter with AV block:* P waves have flutter morphology with fixed relationship of flutter waves to QRS complexes.

- COMPLETE AV BLOCK WITH JUNCTIONAL RHYTHM

    Sinus P rate is equal to or greater than QRS rate with AV dissociation.

R-R INTERVAL	REGULAR
QRS RATE	DECREASED
QRS DURATION	NORMAL

(See Figs. 22–24.)

R-R INTERVAL	REGULAR
QRS RATE	DECREASED
QRS DURATION	NORMAL

Figure 22.

Top tracing:
>Sinus bradycardia
>Ventricular rate = 50/min
>Atrial rate = 50/min

Second tracing:
>Ectopic atrial bradycardia
>Ventricular rate = 50/min
>Atrial rate = 50/min

Third tracing:
>Junctional rhythm with AV dissociation
>Ventricular rate = 50/min
>Atrial rate = 48/min
>Conduction does not occur from ventricles to atria.

Bottom tracing:
>Junctional rhythm
>Ventricular rate = 50/min
>Atrial rate = 50/min
>Retrograde conduction is intact with inverted P waves following each QRS complex.

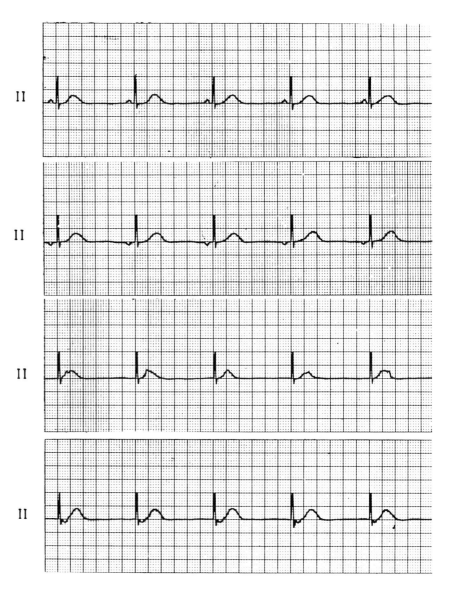

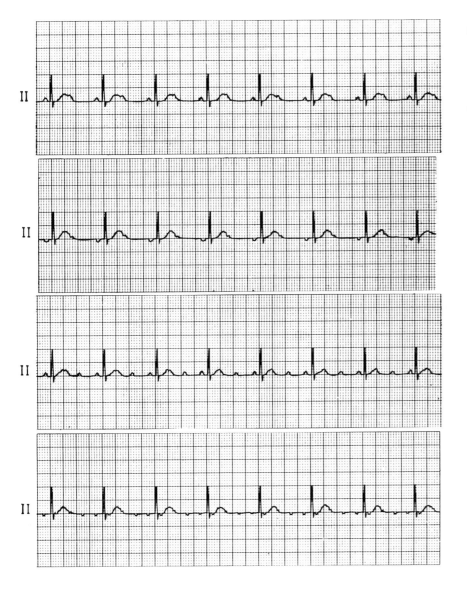

Figure 23.

Top tracing:
    Sinus rhythm with second degree AV block (2 : 1)
    Ventricular rate = 50/min
    Atrial rate = 100/min
    Every other P wave is followed by a QRS complex; when AV block is 2 : 1, it is not possible to determine if this is type I or type II second degree AV block.

Second tracing:
    Atrial rhythm with second degree AV block (2 : 1)
    Ventricular rate = 50/min
    Atrial rate = 100/min

Third tracing:
    Sinus rhythm (rapid rate) with fixed type II second degree AV block (3 : 1)
    Ventricular rate = 50/min
    Atrial rate = 150/min

Bottom tracing:
    Supraventricular tachycardia with fixed type II second degree AV block (5 : 1)
    Ventricular rate = 50/min
    Atrial rate = 250/min

R-R INTERVAL   REGULAR
QRS RATE   DECREASED
QRS DURATION NORMAL

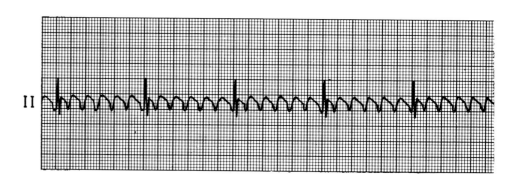

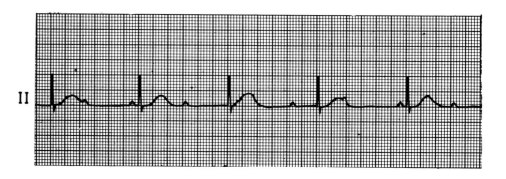

R-R INTERVAL	REGULAR
QRS RATE	DECREASED
QRS DURATION	NORMAL

Figure 24.

Top tracing:

Atrial flutter with fixed type II second degree AV
block (6 : 1)
Ventricular rate = 50/min
Atrial rate = 300/min

Bottom tracing:

Complete AV block with AV dissociation and junc-
tional rhythm
Ventricular rate = 50/min
Atrial rate = 85/min

R-R INTERVAL	REGULAR
QRS RATE	DECREASED
QRS DURATION	PROLONGED

(See Figs. 25–27.)

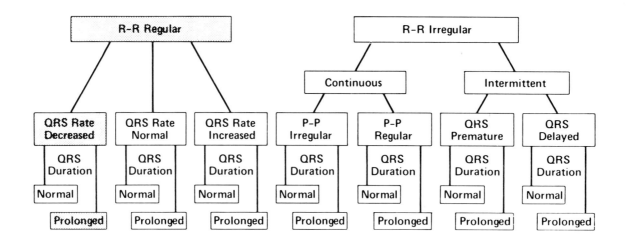

- SINUS BRADYCARDIA WITH ABERRATION

  P wave precedes each QRS complex with a normal P wave axis.

- ECTOPIC ATRIAL BRADYCARDIA WITH ABERRATION

  P wave precedes each QRS complex with an abnormal P wave axis.

- JUNCTIONAL RHYTHM WITH ABERRATION OR
  IDIOVENTRICULAR RHYTHM

  P rate is less than QRS rate with AV dissociation, or "retrograde" P wave follows some or all QRS complexes with R-P interval < 0.30 sec.

- SUPRAVENTRICULAR RHYTHM WITH FIXED TYPE II
  SECOND DEGREE AV BLOCK AND ABERRATION

  P rate is a multiple of QRS rate with a fixed relationship of P waves to QRS complexes (see supraventricular rhythm with fixed type II second degree AV block, page 37).

- COMPLETE AV BLOCK WITH VENTRICULAR RHYTHM

  P rate is equal to or greater than QRS rate with AV dissociation.

R-R INTERVAL	REGULAR
QRS RATE	DECREASED
QRS DURATION	PROLONGED

(See Figs. 25–27.)

R-R INTERVAL	**REGULAR**
QRS RATE	**DECREASED**
QRS DURATION	**PROLONGED**

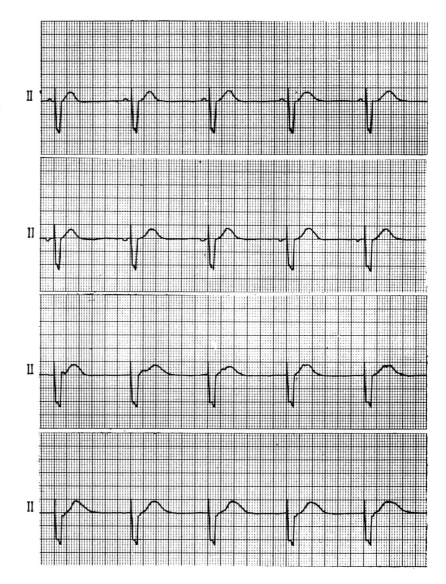

Figure 25.

Top tracing:

　Sinus bradycardia with CRBBB

　Ventricular rate = 50/min

　Atrial rate = 50/min

Second tracing:

　Ectopic atrial bradycardia with CRBBB

　Ventricular rate = 50/min

　Atrial rate = 50/min

Third tracing:

　Junctional rhythm with CRBBB or idioventricular rhythm with AV dissociation (it is impossible to distinguish between these on surface ECG).

　Ventricular rate = 50/min

　Atrial rate = 48/min

　Conduction does not occur from ventricles to atria.

Bottom tracing:

　Junctional rhythm with CRBBB or idioventricular rhythm (inverted P waves following each QRS complex).

　Ventricular rate = 50/min

　Atrial rate = 50/min

　Retrograde conduction is intact with inverted P waves following each QRS complex.

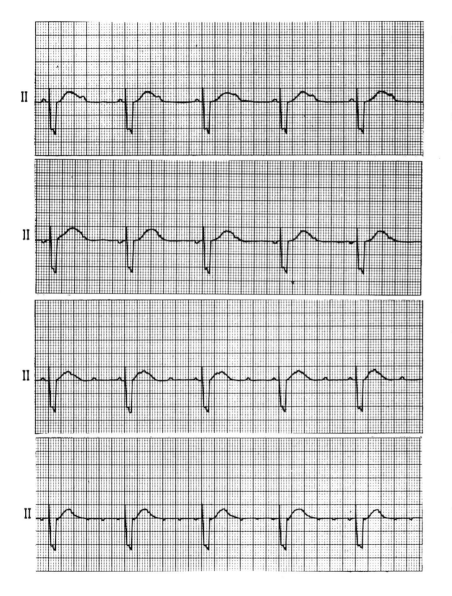

R-R INTERVAL   REGULAR
QRS RATE   DECREASED
QRS DURATION   PROLONGED

Figure 26.

Top tracing:

    Sinus rhythm with second degree AV block (2 : 1) and CRBBB

    Ventricular rate = 50/min

    Atrial rate = 100/min

    Every other P wave is followed by a QRS complex; when AV block is 2 : 1, it is not possible to determine if this is type I or type II second degree AV block.

Second tracing:

    Atrial rhythm with second degree AV block (2 : 1) and CRBBB

    Ventricular rate = 50/min

    Atrial rate = 100/min

Third tracing:

    Sinus rhythm (rapid rate) with fixed type II second degree AV block (3 : 1) and CRBBB

    Ventricular rate = 50/min

    Atrial rate = 150/min

Bottom tracing:

    Supraventricular tachycardia with fixed type II second degree AV block (5 : 1) and CRBBB

    Ventricular rate = 50/min

    Atrial rate = 250/min

R-R INTERVAL	**REGULAR**
QRS RATE	**DECREASED**
QRS DURATION	**PROLONGED**

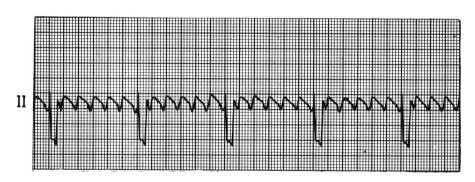

II

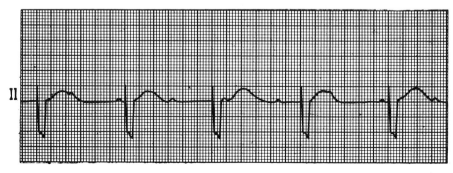

II

R-R INTERVAL	**REGULAR**
QRS RATE	**DECREASED**
QRS DURATION	**PROLONGED**

Figure 27.

Top tracing:

   Atrial flutter with fixed type II second degree AV block (6 : 1) and CRBBB
   Ventricular rate = 50/min
   Atrial rate = 300/min

Bottom tracing:

   Complete AV block with AV dissociation and junctional rhythm with CRBBB or idioventricular rhythm
   Ventricular rate = 50/min
   Atrial rate = 85/min

R-R INTERVAL   REGULAR
QRS RATE   NORMAL
QRS DURATION   NORMAL

(See Figs. 28–30.)

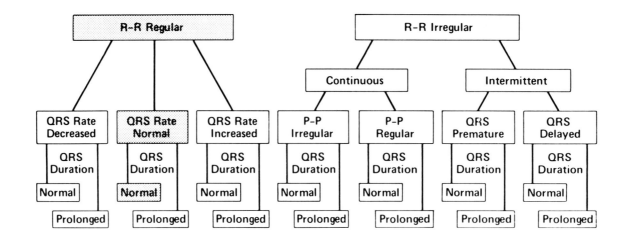

- SINUS RHYTHM

  P wave precedes each QRS complex with a normal P wave axis.

- ECTOPIC ATRIAL RHYTHM

  P wave precedes each QRS complex with an abnormal P wave axis.

- ACCELERATED JUNCTIONAL RHYTHM

  Sinus P rate less than QRS rate with AV dissociation, or no P waves are visible, or retrograde P wave follows some or all QRS complexes.

- SUPRAVENTRICULAR RHYTHM WITH FIXED TYPE II
  SECOND DEGREE AV BLOCK

  P rate is a multiple of QRS rate with a fixed relationship of P waves to QRS complexes (see supraventricular rhythm with fixed type II second degree AV block, page 37).

R-R INTERVAL	REGULAR
QRS RATE	NORMAL
QRS DURATION	NORMAL

R-R INTERVAL	REGULAR
QRS RATE	NORMAL
QRS DURATION	NORMAL

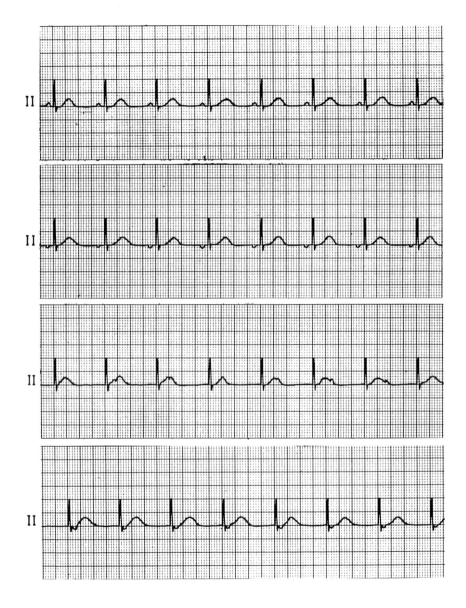

Figure 28.

Top tracing:
> Sinus rhythm
> Ventricular rate = 75/min
> Atrial rate = 75/min

Second tracing:
> Ectopic atrial rhythm
> Ventricular rate = 75/min
> Atrial rate = 75/min

Third tracing:
> Accelerated junctional rhythm with AV dissociation
> Ventricular rate = 75/min
> Atrial rate = 71/min
> Conduction does not occur from ventricles to atria.

Bottom tracing:
> Accelerated junctional rhythm
> Ventricular rate = 75/min
> Atrial rate = 75/min
> Retrograde conduction is intact with inverted P waves following each QRS complex.

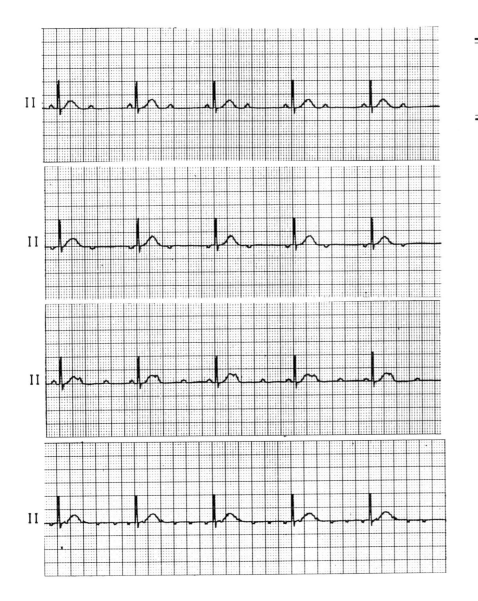

Figure 29.

Top tracing:
Sinus rhythm with second degree AV block (2 : 1)
Ventricular rate = 75/min
Atrial rate = 150/min
Every other P wave is followed by a QRS complex; when AV block is 2 : 1, it is not possible to determine if this is type I or type II second degree AV block.

Second tracing:
Atrial rhythm with second degree AV block (2 : 1)
Ventricular rate = 75/min
Atrial rate = 150/min

Third tracing:
Sinus tachycardia with fixed type II second degree AV block (3 : 1)
Ventricular rate = 75/min
Atrial rate = 225/min

Bottom tracing:
Supraventricular tachycardia with fixed type II second degree AV block (4 : 1)
Ventricular rate = 75/min
Atrial rate = 300/min

R-R INTERVAL	REGULAR
QRS RATE	NORMAL
QRS DURATION	NORMAL

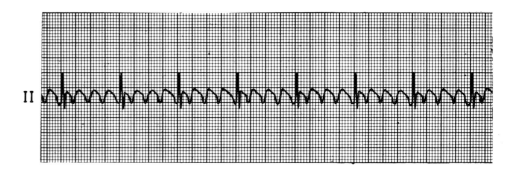

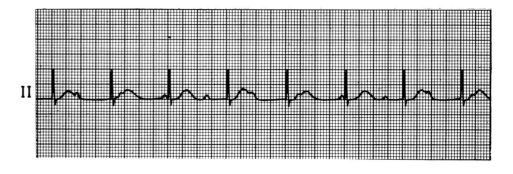

R-R INTERVAL	REGULAR
QRS RATE	NORMAL
QRS DURATION	NORMAL

Figure 30.

Top tracing:

Atrial flutter with fixed type II second degree AV
block (4 : 1)
Ventricular rate = 75/min
Atrial rate = 300/min

Bottom tracing:

Complete AV block with AV dissociation and accel-
erated junctional rhythm
Ventricular rate = 75/min
Atrial rate = 100/min

R-R INTERVAL   REGULAR
QRS RATE   NORMAL
QRS DURATION   PROLONGED

(See Figs. 31–33.)

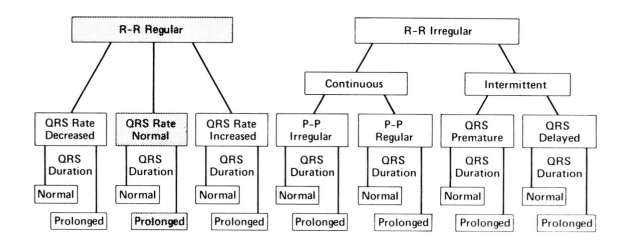

- SINUS RHYTHM WITH ABERRATION

  P wave precedes each QRS complex with a normal P wave axis.

- ECTOPIC ATRIAL RHYTHM WITH ABERRATION

  P wave precedes each QRS complex with an abnormal P wave axis.

- ACCELERATED JUNCTIONAL RHYTHM WITH
  ABERRATION OR VENTRICULAR TACHYCARDIA

  Sinus P rate is less than QRS rate with AV dissociation, or no P wave is visible, or retrograde P wave follows some or all QRS complexes.

- SUPRAVENTRICULAR RHYTHM WITH ABERRATION
  AND FIXED TYPE II SECOND DEGREE AV BLOCK

  P rate is a multiple of QRS rate with a fixed relationship of P waves to QRS complexes (see supraventricular rhythm with fixed type II second degree AV block, page 37).

R-R INTERVAL	REGULAR
QRS RATE	NORMAL
QRS DURATION	PROLONGED

R-R INTERVAL   REGULAR
QRS RATE   NORMAL
QRS DURATION   PROLONGED

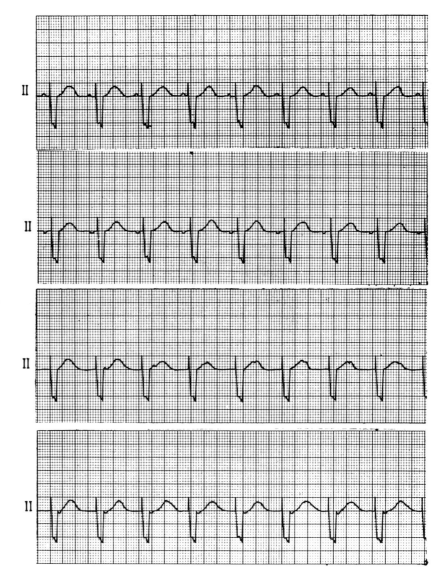

Figure 31.

Top tracing:
Sinus rhythm with CRBBB
Ventricular rate = 85/min
Atrial rate = 85/min

Second tracing:
Ectopic atrial rhythm with CRBBB
Ventricular rate = 85/min
Atrial rate = 85/min

Third tracing:
Accelerated junctional rhythm with CRBBB or ventricular tachycardia with AV dissociation (it is impossible to distinguish between these on surface ECG).
Ventricular rate = 85/min
Atrial rate = 80/min
Conduction does not occur from ventricles to atria.

Bottom tracing:
Accelerated junctional rhythm with CRBBB or ventricular tachycardia
Ventricular rate = 85/min
Atrial rate = 85/min
Retrograde conduction is intact with inverted P waves following each QRS complex.

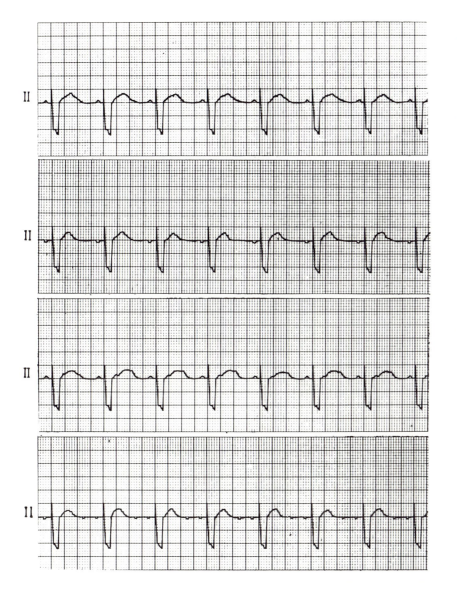

II

II

II

II

R-R INTERVAL   REGULAR
QRS RATE   NORMAL
QRS DURATION PROLONGED

Figure 32.

Top tracing:
Sinus rhythm with second degree AV block (2 : 1) and CRBBB
Ventricular rate = 75/min
Atrial rate = 150/min
Every other P wave is followed by a QRS complex; when AV block is 2 : 1, it is not possible to determine if this is type I or type II second degree AV block.

Second tracing:
Atrial rhythm with second degree AV block (2 : 1) and CRBBB
Ventricular rate = 75/min
Atrial rate = 150/min

Third tracing:
Sinus tachycardia with fixed type II second degree AV block (3 : 1) and CRBBB
Ventricular rate = 75/min
Atrial rate = 225/min

Bottom tracing:
Supraventricular tachycardia with fixed type II second degree AV block (4 : 1) and CRBBB
Ventricular rate = 75/min
Atrial rate = 300/min

R-R INTERVAL   REGULAR
QRS RATE   NORMAL
QRS DURATION PROLONGED

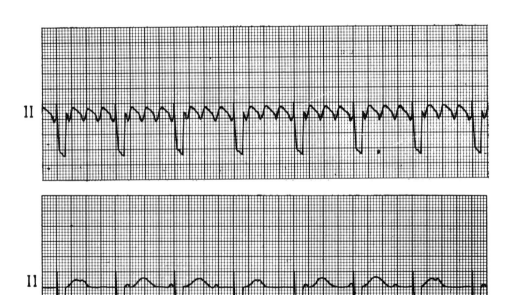

R-R INTERVAL	REGULAR
QRS RATE	NORMAL
QRS DURATION	PROLONGED

Figure 33.

Top tracing:
    Atrial flutter with fixed type II second degree AV
    block (4 : 1) and CRBBB
    Ventricular rate = 75/min
    Atrial rate = 300/min

Bottom tracing:
    Complete AV block with AV dissociation and accel-
    erated junctional rhythm with CRBBB or ventricu-
    lar tachycardia
    Ventricular rate = 75/min
    Atrial rate = 100/min

R-R INTERVAL	REGULAR
QRS RATE	INCREASED
QRS DURATION	NORMAL

(See Figs. 34–36.)

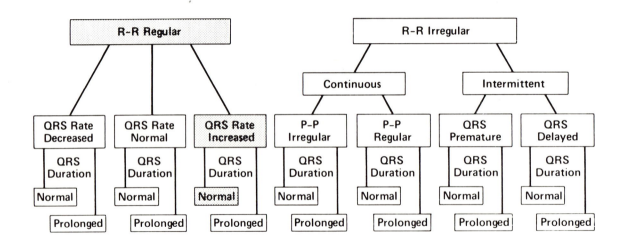

- SINUS TACHYCARDIA (1 : 1 CONDUCTION)

     P wave precedes each QRS complex with a normal P wave axis and P rate ≤ 230/min.

- ECTOPIC ATRIAL TACHYCARDIA (1 : 1 CONDUCTION)

     P wave precedes each QRS complex with an abnormal P wave axis.

- SUPRAVENTRICULAR TACHYCARDIA (1 : 1
  CONDUCTION)

     P wave is visible between some or all QRS complexes with constant PR interval, or no P wave is visible, or sinus P rate is less than the QRS rate with AV dissociation.

- SUPRAVENTRICULAR TACHYCARDIA WITH FIXED
  TYPE II SECOND DEGREE AV BLOCK

     P rate is a multiple of QRS rate with a fixed relationship of P waves to QRS complexes.

- ATRIAL FLUTTER WITH FIXED TYPE II
  SECOND DEGREE AV BLOCK

     P waves have flutter morphology with a fixed relationship of flutter waves to QRS complexes.

R-R INTERVAL   REGULAR
QRS RATE   INCREASED
QRS DURATION   NORMAL

(See Figs. 34–36.)

R-R INTERVAL	**REGULAR**
QRS RATE	**INCREASED**
QRS DURATION	**NORMAL**

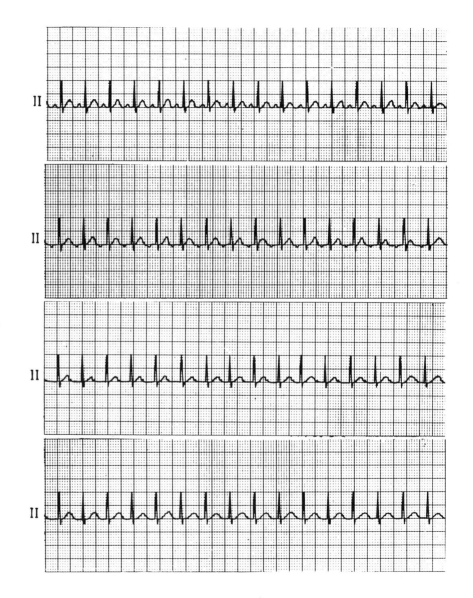

Figure 34.

Top tracing:
> Sinus tachycardia
> Ventricular rate = 160/min
> Atrial rate = 160/min
> P axis 0°–90°, PR interval 0.12 sec

Second tracing:
> Ectopic atrial tachycardia
> (This is a type of supraventricular tachycardia. In supraventricular tachycardia, P waves may be present or absent and the PR interval may be normal or prolonged. In this and the next five tracings, some of the various morphologies of supraventricular tachycardia are presented.)
> Ventricular rate = 160/min
> Atrial rate = 160/min
> P axis 270°–359°, PR interval 0.12 sec

Third tracing:
> Supraventricular tachycardia
> Ventricular rate = 160/min
> Atrial rate = 160/min
> P axis 270°–359°, PR interval 0.20 sec

Bottom tracing:
> Supraventricular tachycardia
> Ventricular rate = 160/min
> No P waves are visible.

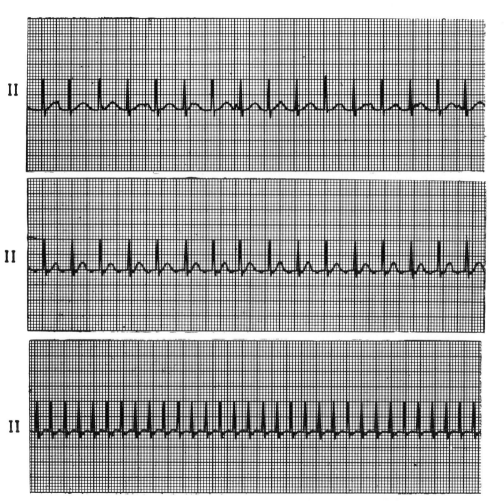

II

II

II

Figure 35.

Top tracing:

Supraventricular tachycardia with AV dissociation
Ventricular rate = 160/min
Atrial rate = 100/min
P axis 0°–90°, PR interval variable
The P waves are from the sinus node depolarizing the atria and the QRS complexes are from the AV junction depolarizing the ventricles.

Middle tracing:

Supraventricular tachycardia with second degree AV block (2 : 1)
Ventricular rate = 160/min
Atrial rate = 320/min
P axis 270°–359°
There are two PR intervals, 0.12 sec and 0.33 sec. From the surface ECG it is not possible to determine which P wave causes the QRS.

Bottom tracing:

Supraventricular tachycardia
This is the same example shown in the middle tracing, but with 1 : 1 conduction.
Ventricular rate = 320/min
Atrial rate = 320/min
P axis 270°–359°, PR interval 0.14 sec
Inverted P waves immediately follow each QRS.

II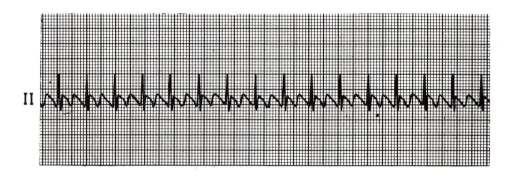

II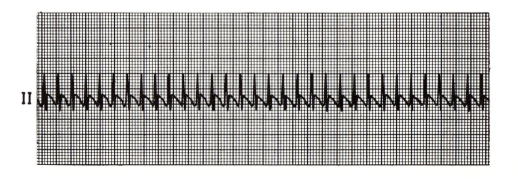

Figure 36.

Top tracing:

    Atrial flutter with second degree AV block (2 : 1)

    Ventricular rate = 160/min

    Atrial rate = 320/min

Bottom tracing:

    Atrial flutter

    This is the same example shown in the top tracing,

    but with 1 : 1 conduction.

    Ventricular rate = 320/min

    Atrial rate = 320/min

R-R INTERVAL   REGULAR
QRS RATE   INCREASED
QRS DURATION   PROLONGED

(See Figs. 37–40.)

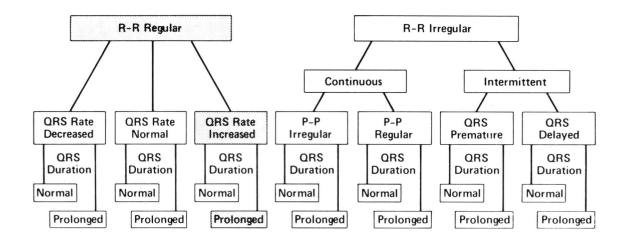

- SINUS TACHYCARDIA (1 : 1 CONDUCTION)
  WITH ABERRATION

  P wave precedes each QRS complex with a normal P wave axis.

- ECTOPIC ATRIAL TACHYCARDIA (1 : 1 CONDUCTION)
  WITH ABERRATION

  P wave precedes each QRS complex with an abnormal P wave axis.

- SUPRAVENTRICULAR TACHYCARDIA (1 : 1
  CONDUCTION) WITH ABERRATION OR VENTRICULAR
  TACHYCARDIA

  P wave is visible between some or all QRS complexes with constant PR interval, or no P wave is visible, or sinus P rate is less than QRS rate with AV dissociation.

- SUPRAVENTRICULAR TACHYCARDIA WITH
  ABERRATION AND FIXED TYPE II SECOND DEGREE AV
  BLOCK

  P rate is a multiple of QRS rate with fixed relationship of P waves to QRS complexes

- ATRIAL FLUTTER WITH ABERRATION AND FIXED
  TYPE II SECOND DEGREE AV BLOCK

  P waves have flutter morphology with a fixed relationship of flutter waves to QRS complexes.

R-R INTERVAL	REGULAR
QRS RATE	INCREASED
QRS DURATION	PROLONGED

(See Figs. 37–40.)

R-R INTERVAL	**REGULAR**
QRS RATE	**INCREASED**
QRS DURATION	**PROLONGED**

Figure 37.

Top tracing:

Sinus tachycardia with CRBBB
Ventricular rate = 160/min
Atrial rate = 160/min
P axis 0°–90°, PR interval 0.12 sec

Second tracing:

Sinus tachycardia with CRBBB
This tracing is the same as the top tracing, except that the T waves have greater amplitude and the P waves are on the downslope of the T waves.
Ventricular rate = 160/min
Atrial rate = 160/min
P axis 0°–90°, PR interval 0.12 sec
This is unlikely to be ventricular tachycardia because the P waves are related to the QRS complexes and the P wave axis is normal.

Third tracing:

Ectopic atrial tachycardia with CRBBB or ventricular tachycardia with 1 : 1 retrograde conduction to the atria
Ventricular rate = 160/min
Atrial rate = 160/min
P axis 270°–359°, PR interval 0.12 sec
The P waves could either originate in the low atrium (from ectopic supraventricular tachycardia) and conduct to the ventricles or could be conducted retrogradely from ventricular tachycardia. It is impossible to distinguish between the two on surface ECG. In children, however, supraventricular tachycardia with aberration is much less common than ventricular tachycardia.

Bottom tracing:

Etopic atrial tachycardia with CRBBB or ventricular tachycardia
This tracing is the same as the third tracing, except that the T waves have greater amplitude and the P waves are on the downslope of the T waves.
Ventricular rate = 160/min
Atrial rate = 160/min
P axis 270°–359°, PR interval 0.12 sec

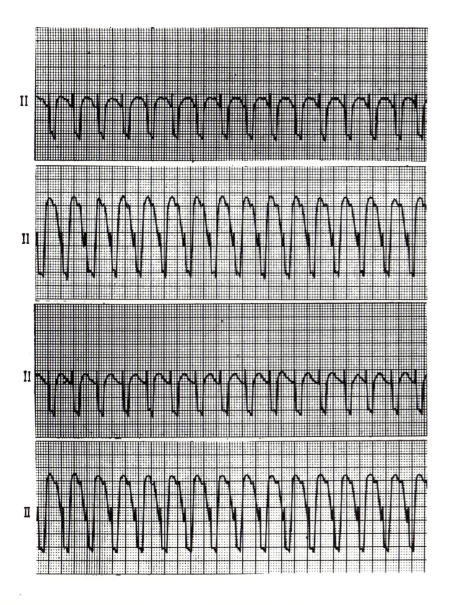

R-R INTERVAL	REGULAR
QRS RATE	INCREASED
QRS DURATION	PROLONGED

R-R INTERVAL	**REGULAR**
QRS RATE	**INCREASED**
QRS DURATION	**PROLONGED**

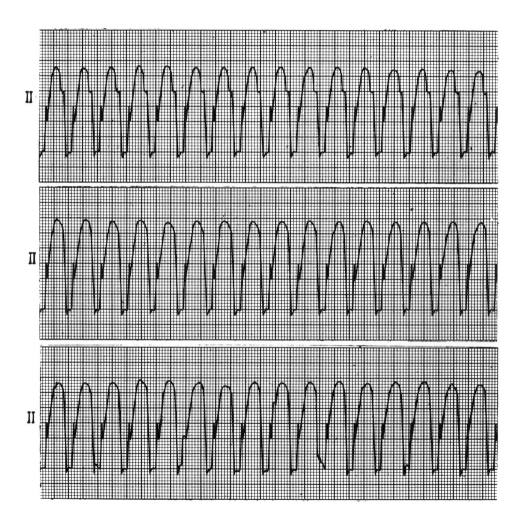

Figure 38.

Top tracing:
Supraventricular tachycardia with CRBBB or ventricular tachycardia
Ventricular rate = 160/min
Atrial rate = 160/min
Inverted P waves are visible on the upstroke of the T waves.
P axis 270°–359°, PR interval 0.24 sec

Second tracing:
Supraventricular tachycardia with CRBBB or ventricular tachycardia
Ventricular rate = 160/min
P waves are not visible consistently.

Bottom tracing:
Supraventricular tachycardia with CRBBB or ventricular tachycardia
There is complete AV dissociation
Ventricular rate = 160/min
Atrial rate = 100/min
P axis 0°–90° (sinus P waves), PR interval variable

Figure 39.

Top tracing:

> Supraventricular tachycardia with CRBBB and second degree AV block (2 : 1)
>
> Ventricular rate = 160/min
>
> Atrial rate = 320/min
>
> P axis 270°–359°
>
> There are two PR intervals, 0.12 sec and 0.32 sec (the P wave with the PR interval of 0.32 sec is concealed in the S wave of the BBB pattern—compare Fig. 38). Ventricular tachycardia would be an unlikely diagnosis because the P waves and QRS complexes are related, with two P waves for each QRS complex.

Bottom tracing:

> Supraventricular tachycardia with CRBBB or ventricular tachycardia
>
> This is the same example as the top tracing, except with 1 : 1 conduction.
>
> Ventricular rate = 320/min
>
> Atrial rate = 320/min
>
> P axis 270°–359°, PR interval 0.32 sec
>
> It is impossible to distinguish between the two on surface ECG, except that this is an uncommonly high rate for ventricular tachycardia.

II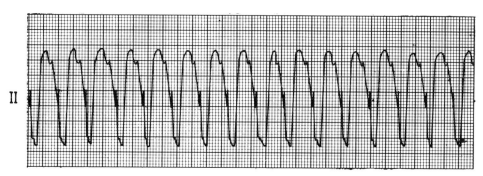

II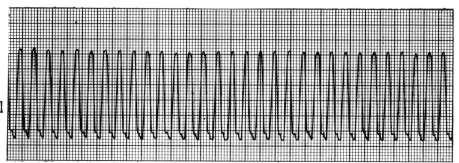

R-R INTERVAL REGULAR
QRS RATE INCREASED
QRS DURATION PROLONGED

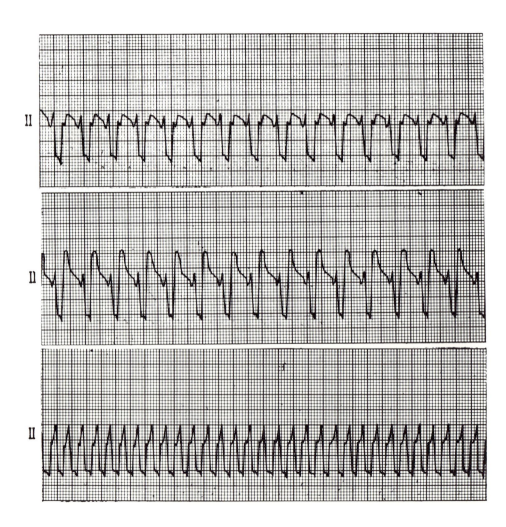

Figure 40.

Top tracing:

Atrial flutter with second degree AV block (2 : 1) and CRBBB

Ventricular rate = 160/min

Atrial rate = 320/min

P axis 270°–359°

The sawtooth baseline is partially concealed. This could be mistaken for supraventricular tachycardia with CRBBB or for ventricular tachycardia.

Middle tracing:

Atrial flutter with second degree AV block (2 : 1) and CRBBB

This is the same example as the top tracing, except that the T waves have greater amplitude.

Ventricular rate = 160/min

Atrial rate = 320/min

The sawtooth baseline is concealed. This could be mistaken for supraventricular tachycardia with CRBBB or ventricular tachycardia. An esophageal lead showing two atrial depolarizations for each QRS complex would help with the diagnosis.

Bottom tracing:

Atrial flutter with CRBBB or ventricular tachycardia

This is the same example as the top and middle tracings, except with 1 : 1 conduction.

Ventricular rate = 320/min

Atrial rate = 320/min

The sawtooth appearance is apparent between QRS complexes, but this could be mistaken for ventricular tachycardia. This is a very common rate for atrial flutter and an uncommon rate for ventricular tachycardia.

R-R INTERVAL	IRREGULAR
R-R INTERVAL	VARIES CONTINUOUSLY
P-P INTERVAL	IRREGULAR
QRS DURATION	NORMAL

(See Fig. 41.)

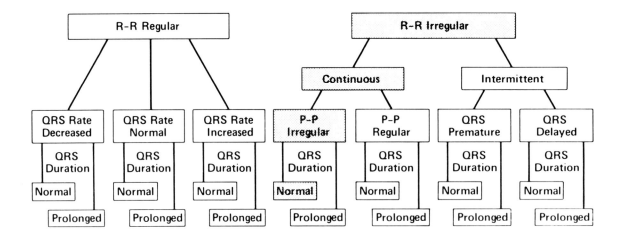

- SINUS ARRHYTHMIA

1. P wave axis may vary between 0°–90°.
2. P wave precedes each QRS complex with variation in PR interval ≤ 0.02 sec.
3. R-R interval prolongs and shortens cyclically with respiration.

(Sinus, atrial, and junctional pacemakers are all under vagal influence and so the rate of rhythms originating from all these sites can vary cyclically. Therefore, sinus, atrial, and junctional rhythm can all have "sinus arrhythmia.")

- WANDERING PACEMAKER

1. P wave axis continually changes—sinus, atrial, junctional.
2. QRS complexes are related to all P waves; either P wave precedes QRS (sinus, atrial origin of P wave) or follows QRS (junctional origin of P wave). P waves may not be visible following junctional beats.

- ATRIAL FIBRILLATION

1. Atrial depolarizations have fibrillation morphology.
2. "Irregularly irregular"—R-R intervals are all usually different.

R-R INTERVAL	**IRREGULAR**
R-R INTERVAL	**VARIES CONTINUOUSLY**
P-P INTERVAL	**IRREGULAR**
QRS DURATION	**NORMAL**

(See Fig. 41.)

R-R INTERVAL   IRREGULAR
R-R INTERVAL   VARIES CONTINUOUSLY
P-P INTERVAL   IRREGULAR
QRS DURATION NORMAL

Figure 41.

Top tracing:

Sinus arrhythmia
Ventricular rate—variable (R-R interval = 0.48–0.92 sec)
Atrial rate—variable (P-P interval = 0.50–0.88 sec)
P axis—slight variation (45°–90°)
PR interval—slight variation (0.10–0.12 sec)
Inspiration began at the left side of the tracing and the patient breathed approximately every 3 sec (20/min).

Middle tracing:

Wandering pacemaker
Ventricular rate—variable (R-R interval = 0.48–0.92 sec)
Atrial rate—variable (P-P interval = 0.45–1.72 sec)
P axis—variable, when P wave present (0°–359°)
PR interval—slight variation when P wave present (0.10–0.12 sec)

Bottom tracing:

Atrial fibrillation
Ventricular rate—variable (R-R interval = 0.44–1.06 sec); no two R-R intervals are the same.
Atrial rate—fibrillation

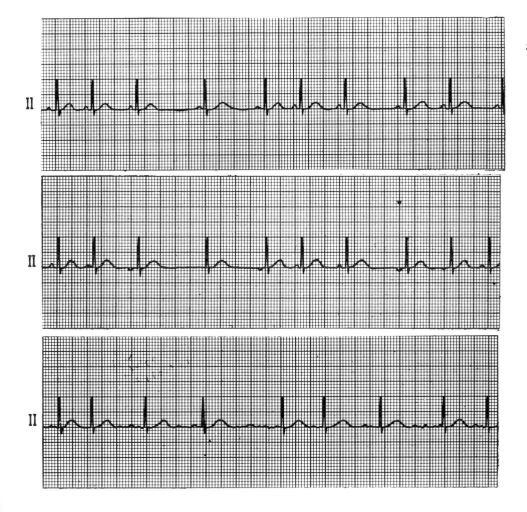

R-R INTERVAL	IRREGULAR
R-R INTERVAL	VARIES CONTINUOUSLY
P-P INTERVAL	IRREGULAR
QRS DURATION	NORMAL

R-R INTERVAL	IRREGULAR
R-R INTERVAL	VARIES CONTINUOUSLY
P-P INTERVAL	IRREGULAR
QRS DURATION	PROLONGED

(See Fig. 42.)

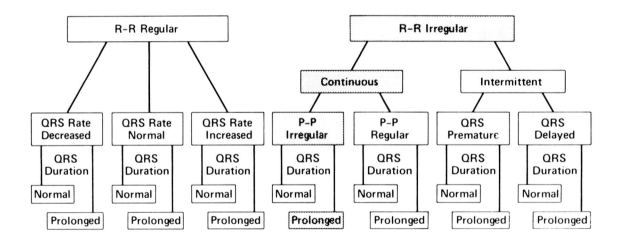

- SINUS ARRHYTHMIA WITH ABERRATION

1. P wave axis may vary between 0°–90°.
2. P wave precedes each QRS complex with variation in PR interval < 0.02 sec.
3. R-R interval prolongs and shortens cyclically with respiration.

(Sinus, atrial, and junctional pacemakers are all under vagal influence and so the rate of rhythms originating from these sites can vary cyclically. Therefore, sinus, atrial, and junctional rhythm can all have "sinus arrhythmia.")

- WANDERING PACEMAKER WITH ABERRATION

1. P wave axis continually changes—sinus, atrial, junctional.
2. QRS complexes are related to all P waves; either the P wave precedes QRS (sinus, atrial origin of P wave) or follows QRS (junctional origin of P wave).

- ATRIAL FIBRILLATION WITH ABERRATION

1. Atrial depolarizations have fibrillation morphology.
2. "Irregularly irregular"—R-R intervals are usually different.

R-R INTERVAL	**IRREGULAR**
R-R INTERVAL	**VARIES CONTINUOUSLY**
P-P INTERVAL	**IRREGULAR**
QRS DURATION	**PROLONGED**

(See Fig. 42.)

R-R INTERVAL	**IRREGULAR**
R-R INTERVAL	**VARIES CONTINUOUSLY**
P-P INTERVAL	**IRREGULAR**
QRS DURATION	**PROLONGED**

Figure 42.

Top tracing:

Sinus arrhythmia with CRBBB
Ventricular rate—variable (R-R interval = 0.48–0.92 sec)
Atrial rate—variable (P-P interval = 0.50–0.88 sec)
P axis—slight variation (45°–90°)
PR interval—slight variation (0.10–0.12 sec)
Inspiration began at the left side of the tracing and the patient breathed approximately every 3 sec (20/min).

Middle tracing:

Wandering pacemaker with CRBBB
Ventricular rate—variable (R-R interval = 0.48–0.92 sec)
Atrial rate—variable (P-P interval = 0.45–1.72 sec)
P axis—variable, when P wave present (0°–359°)
PR interval—slight variation, when P wave present (0.10–0.12 sec)

Bottom tracing:

Atrial fibrillation with CRBBB
Ventricular rate—variable (R-R interval = 0.44–1.06 sec); no two R-R intervals are the same.
Atrial rate—fibrillation

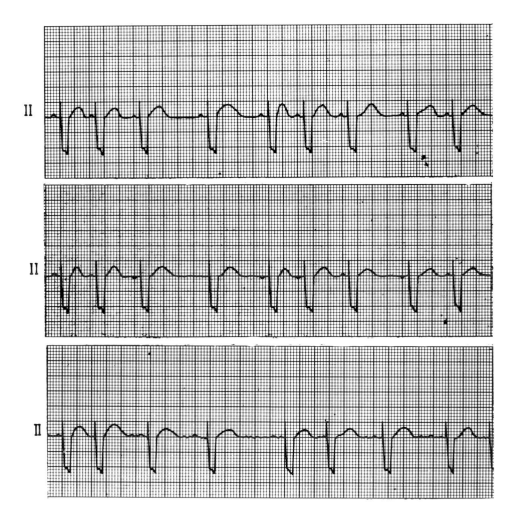

R-R INTERVAL	IRREGULAR
R-R INTERVAL	VARIES CONTINUOUSLY
P-P INTERVAL	IRREGULAR
QRS DURATION	PROLONGED

R-R INTERVAL	IRREGULAR
R-R INTERVAL	VARIES CONTINUOUSLY
P-P INTERVAL	REGULAR
QRS DURATION	NORMAL

(See Fig. 43.)

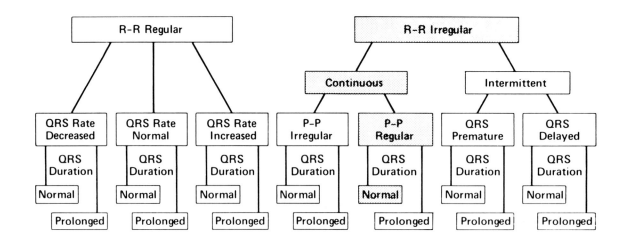

- SUPRAVENTRICULAR RHYTHM WITH VARYING TYPE II
  SECOND DEGREE AV BLOCK

1. R-R interval is a varying multiple of the P-P interval.
2. All R waves are preceded by a P wave with the same PR interval.

- SUPRAVENTRICULAR RHYTHM WITH TYPE I SECOND
  DEGREE AV BLOCK (WENCKEBACH)

1. R-R interval progressively shortens.
2. PR interval progressively lengthens until a single P wave is not followed by a QRS
   complex.

Note. See supraventricular rhythm with fixed type II second degree AV block, page
37.

R-R INTERVAL	**IRREGULAR**
R-R INTERVAL	**VARIES CONTINUOUSLY**
P-P INTERVAL	**REGULAR**
QRS DURATION	**NORMAL**

(See Fig. 43.)

R-R INTERVAL	IRREGULAR
R-R INTERVAL	VARIES CONTINUOUSLY
P-P INTERVAL	REGULAR
QRS DURATION	PROLONGED

Figure 43.

Top tracing:
> Sinus tachycardia with varying type II second degree AV block (3 : 1, 2 : 1, 1 : 1 conduction)
> Ventricular rate—variable (R-R interval = 0.28–0.88 sec)
> Atrial rate = 214/min
> P axis 0°–90°
> PR interval = 0.12 sec on conducted beats

Second tracing:
> Atrial flutter with varying type II second degree AV block (3 : 1, 2 : 1, 1 : 1 conduction)
> Ventricular rate—variable (R-R interval = 0.20–0.80 sec)
> Atrial rate = 300/min

Third tracing:
> Sinus tachycardia with type I second degree AV block (5 : 4 Wenckebach)
> Ventricular rate—variable (R-R intervals progressively shorten within a group of four QRS complexes. From beginning of tracing—0.48, 0.40, 0.38 sec. Then the blocked P wave causes a pause of 0.74 sec and the cycle begins again.)
> Atrial rate = 167/min
> P axis 0°–90°
> PR interval—variable (PR intervals progressively lengthen within a group of four QRS complexes. From beginning of tracing—0.12, 0.24, 0.28, 0.30 sec. Then there is a P wave without a following QRS complex and the cycle begins again.)

Bottom tracing:
> Atrial flutter with type I second degree AV block (5 : 4 Wenckebach)
> Ventricular rate—variable (R-R intervals progres-

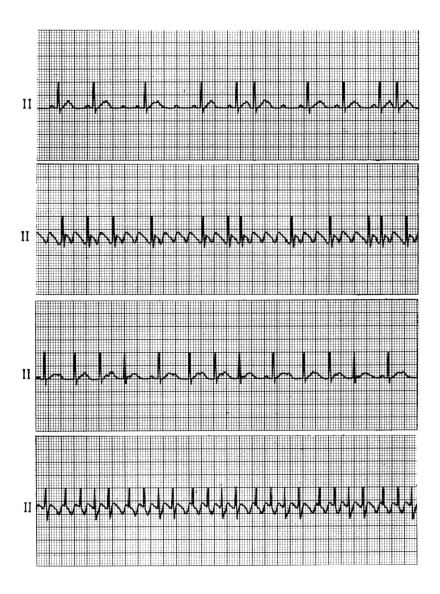

II

R-R INTERVAL	IRREGULAR
R-R INTERVAL	VARIES CONTINUOUSLY
P-P INTERVAL	REGULAR
QRS DURATION	PROLONGED

sively shorten within a group of four QRS complexes. From beginning of tracing—0.32, 0.24, 0.22 sec. The blocked flutter wave causes a pause of 0.22 sec and the cycle begins again.)

Atrial rate = 300/min

Flutter-R interval—variable (Flutter-R intervals progressively lengthen within a group of four QRS complexes. From beginning of tracing—0.12, 0.24, 0.28, 0.30 sec. Then there is a flutter wave without a following QRS complex and the cycle begins again. Flutter waves begin on each dark line every 0.20 sec.)

Note. All supraventricular rhythms can have second degree AV block (see supraventricular rhythm with fixed type II second degree AV block, page 37), although only sinus tachycardia and atrial flutter are shown here.

R-R INTERVAL	IRREGULAR
R-R INTERVAL	VARIES CONTINUOUSLY
P-P INTERVAL	REGULAR
QRS DURATION	PROLONGED

(See Fig. 44.)

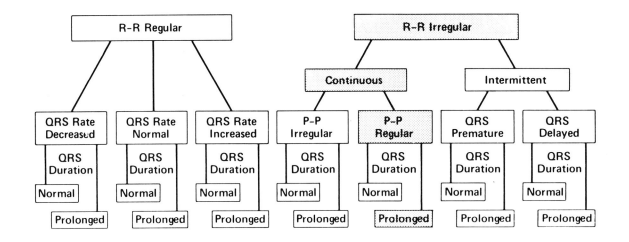

- SUPRAVENTRICULAR RHYTHM WITH ABERRATION
  AND VARYING TYPE II SECOND DEGREE AV BLOCK

1. R-R interval is a varying multiple of P-P interval.
2. All R waves are preceded by a P wave with the same PR interval.

- SUPRAVENTRICULAR RHYTHM WITH ABERRATION
  AND TYPE I SECOND DEGREE AV BLOCK
  (WENCKEBACH)

1. R-R interval progressively shortens.
2. PR interval progressively lengthens until a single P wave is not followed by a QRS complex.

Note. See supraventricular rhythm with fixed type II second degree AV block, page 37.

R-R INTERVAL	IRREGULAR
R-R INTERVAL	VARIES CONTINUOUSLY
P-P INTERVAL	REGULAR
QRS DURATION	PROLONGED

R-R INTERVAL	IRREGULAR
R-R INTERVAL	VARIES CONTINUOUSLY
P-P INTERVAL	REGULAR
QRS DURATION	PROLONGED

Figure 44.

Top tracing:

Sinus tachycardia with varying type II second degree AV block (3 : 1, 2 : 1, 1 : 1 conduction) and CRBBB

Ventricular rate—variable (R-R interval = 0.28–0.88 sec)

Atrial rate = 214/min

P axis 0°–90°

PR interval = 0.12 sec on conducted beats (P waves are on the upstroke of all T waves.)

Second tracing:

Atrial flutter with varying type II second degree AV block (3 : 1, 2 : 1, 1 : 1 conduction) and CRBBB

Ventricular rate—variable (R-R interval = 0.20–0.80 sec)

Atrial rate = 300/min

Third tracing:

Sinus tachycardia with type I second degree AV block (5 : 4 Wenckebach) and CRBBB

Ventricular rate—variable (R-R intervals progressively shorten within a group of four QRS complexes. From beginning of tracing—0.48, 0.40, 0.38 sec. Then the blocked P wave causes a pause of 0.74 sec and the cycle begins again.)

Atrial rate = 167/min

P axis 0°–90°

PR interval—variable (PR intervals progressively lengthen within a group of four QRS complexes. From beginning of tracing—0.12, 0.24, 0.28, 0.30 sec. Then there is a P wave without a following QRS complex and the cycle begins again.) The P waves cause the various irregularities in the QRS complexes and T waves.

Bottom tracing:

Atrial flutter with type I second degree AV block (5 : 4 Wenckebach) and CRBBB

Ventricular rate—variable (R-R intervals progressively shorten within a group of four QRS complexes. From beginning of tracing—0.32, 0.24, 0.22 sec. The blocked flutter wave causes a pause of 0.22 sec and the cycle begins again.)

Flutter waves are not visible, but the diagnosis may be inferred from the rate and pattern of the QRS complexes. The atrial rate is inferred to be 300/min.

Note. All supraventricular rhythms can have second degree AV block (see supraventricular rhythm with fixed type II second degree AV block, page 37), although only sinus tachycardia and atrial flutter are shown here.

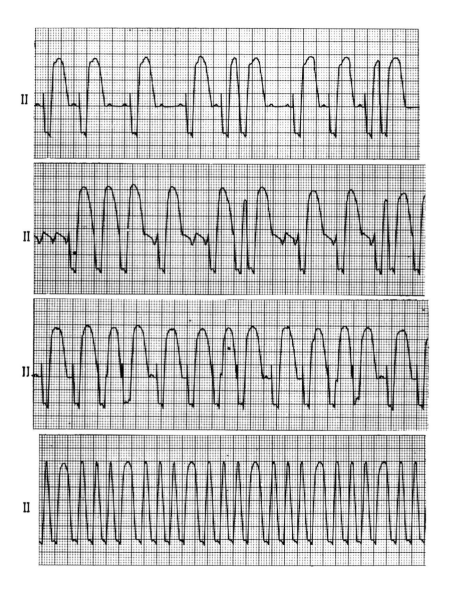

R-R INTERVAL	**IRREGULAR**
R-R INTERVAL	**VARIES CONTINUOUSLY**
P-P INTERVAL	**REGULAR**
QRS DURATION	**PROLONGED**

**BASIC R-R INTERVAL
REGULAR, BUT INTERRUPTED
INTERMITTENTLY**

**IRREGULAR R-R INTERVAL
SHORT (PREMATURE QRS)**

**QRS DURATION OF EARLY COMPLEX
NORMAL**

(See Fig. 45.)

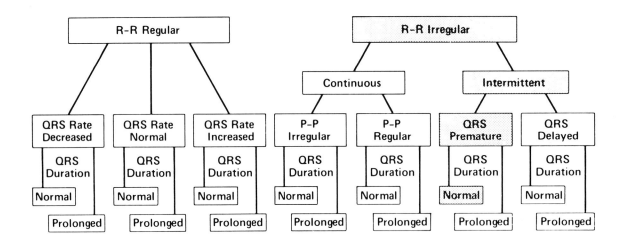

- ECTOPIC ATRIAL OR JUNCTIONAL RHYTHM WITH SINUS CAPTURE

  Early QRS is preceded by a P wave with normal P axis and PR interval < 0.30 sec.

- SINUS, ECTOPIC ATRIAL, OR JUNCTIONAL RHYTHM WITH PREMATURE ATRIAL CONTRAC-TION

  Early QRS is preceded by a P wave with abnormal axis and PR interval < 0.30 sec.

- SINUS, ECTOPIC ATRIAL, OR JUNCTIONAL RHYTHM WITH PREMATURE JUNCTIONAL CON-TRACTION

  Early QRS is not preceded by a P wave.

Note. See supraventricular rhythm with fixed type II second degree AV block, page 37.

BASIC R-R INTERVAL REGULAR, BUT INTERRUPTED INTERMITTENTLY

IRREGULAR R-R INTERVAL SHORT (PREMATURE QRS)

QRS DURATION OF EARLY COMPLEX NORMAL

(See Fig. 45.)

BASIC R-R INTERVAL
REGULAR, BUT INTERRUPTED INTERMITTENTLY

IRREGULAR R-R INTERVAL
SHORT (PREMATURE QRS)

QRS DURATION OF EARLY COMPLEX
NORMAL

Figure 45.

Top tracing:

Junctional rhythm with intermittent sinus capture beats

Atrial rate = 60/min (P-P interval is constant at 1.0 sec.) Sinus bradycardia also is present.

Basic R-R interval regular at 0.80 sec—junctional rhythm

There are two short R-R intervals (0.60 sec) when the third and sixth sinus P waves in the tracing occur at an appropriate time and the AV node is not refractory. Then AV conduction occurs and the P waves are followed closely by QRS complexes. The R-R interval after the fourth QRS is 0.80 sec because the junctional rhythm begins again from the time of the last QRS complex.

Middle tracing:

Sinus rhythm with premature atrial contractions

Basic ventricular and atrial rates = 75/min (R-R and P-P intervals = 0.80 sec). The two short R-R intervals (0.60 sec) occur when a premature P wave (P-P interval = 0.60 sec) with a different P axis con-

ducts to the ventricles. The PR interval of the premature atrial contraction is 0.18 sec, which is longer than the 0.12 sec found in sinus rhythm. The PR interval is longer because the AV node is still relatively refractory when the premature atrial contraction occurs. The R-R interval after the fourth QRS is 0.80 sec (less than compensatory pause) because the premature P wave reset the sinus node.

Bottom tracing:

Sinus rhythm with premature junctional contractions

Basic ventricular and atrial rates = 75/min (R-R and P-P intervals—0.80 sec) The two short R-R intervals (0.60 sec) are caused by identical premature QRS complexes without a preceding P wave, indicating that these are premature junctional contractions. The R-R interval after the fourth QRS is 0.80 sec (less than compensatory pause) because the premature QRS caused the atria to be activated prematurely (retrograde P wave) and reset the sinus node.

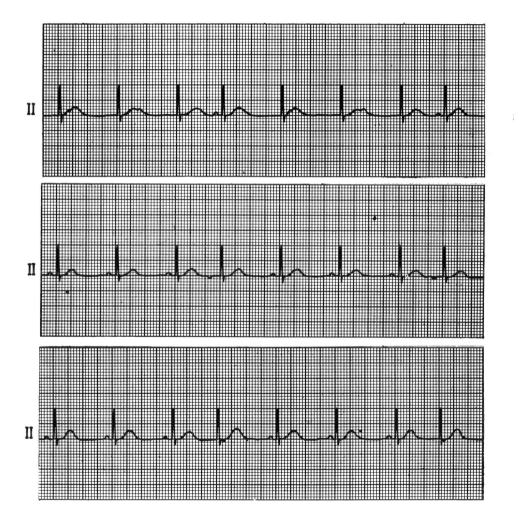

**BASIC R-R INTERVAL
REGULAR, BUT INTERRUPTED
INTERMITTENTLY**

**IRREGULAR R-R INTERVAL
SHORT (PREMATURE QRS)**

**QRS DURATION OF EARLY COMPLEX
NORMAL**

BASIC R-R INTERVAL
REGULAR, BUT INTERRUPTED
INTERMITTENTLY

IRREGULAR R-R INTERVAL
SHORT (PREMATURE QRS)

QRS DURATION OF EARLY COMPLEX
PROLONGED

(See Fig. 46.)

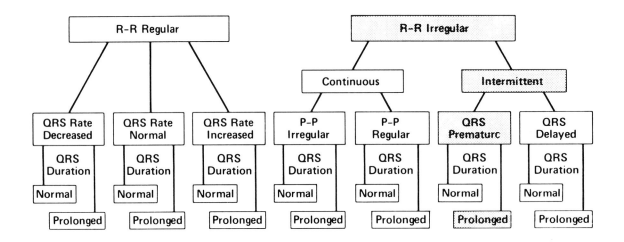

- ECTOPIC ATRIAL OR JUNCTIONAL RHYTHM WITH SINUS CAPTURE AND ABERRATION

    QRS is preceded by a P wave with normal P axis and PR interval < 0.30 sec.

- SINUS, ECTOPIC ATRIAL, OR JUNCTIONAL RHYTHM WITH PREMATURE ATRIAL CONTRACTION AND ABERRATION

    QRS is preceded by an ectopic P wave with abnormal P axis and PR interval < 0.30 sec.

- SINUS, ECTOPIC ATRIAL, OR JUNCTIONAL RHYTHM WITH PREMATURE VENTRICULAR CONTRACTION

    QRS is not preceded by a P wave.

Note. See supraventricular rhythm with fixed type II second degree AV block, page 37.

**BASIC R-R INTERVAL
REGULAR, BUT INTERRUPTED
INTERMITTENTLY**

**IRREGULAR R-R INTERVAL
SHORT (PREMATURE QRS)**

**QRS DURATION OF EARLY COMPLEX
PROLONGED**

(See Fig. 46.)

BASIC R-R INTERVAL
REGULAR, BUT INTERRUPTED
INTERMITTENTLY

IRREGULAR R-R INTERVAL
SHORT (PREMATURE QRS)

QRS DURATION OF EARLY COMPLEX
PROLONGED

Figure 46.

Top tracing:

Junctional rhythm with intermittent sinus capture beats with CRBBB

Atrial rate = 60/min (P-P interval is constant at 1.0 sec). Sinus bradycardia also is present.

Basic R-R interval regular at 0.80 sec—junctional rhythm

There are two short R-R intervals (0.60 sec) when the third and sixth sinus P waves in the tracing occur at an appropriate time and the AV node is not refractory. Then AV conduction occurs and the P waves are followed closely by QRS complexes. The R-R interval after the fourth QRS is 0.80 sec because the junctional rhythm begins again from the time of the last QRS complex.

Middle tracing:

Sinus rhythm with premature atrial contractions and CRBBB

Basic ventricular and atrial rates = 75/min (R-R and P-P intervals = 0.80 sec). The two short R-R intervals (0.60 sec) occur when a premature P wave (P-P interval = 0.60 sec) with a different P axis con-

ducts to the ventricles. The PR interval of the premature atrial contraction is 0.18 sec, which is longer than the 0.12 sec found in sinus rhythm. The PR interval is longer because the AV node is still relatively refractory when the premature atrial contraction occurs. The R-R interval after the fourth QRS is 0.80 sec (less than compensatory pause) because the premature P wave reset the sinus node.

Bottom tracing:

Sinus rhythm with premature ventricular contractions

Basic ventricular and atrial rates = 75/min (R-R and P-P intervals—0.80 sec). The two short R-R intervals (0.60 sec) are caused by premature QRS complexes with prolonged duration without a preceding P wave, indicating that these are premature ventricular contractions. There are retrograde P waves on the upstroke of the T waves. The R-R interval after the fourth QRS is 0.80 sec (less than compensatory pause) because the premature QRS caused the atria to be activated prematurely (retrograde P wave) and reset the sinus node.

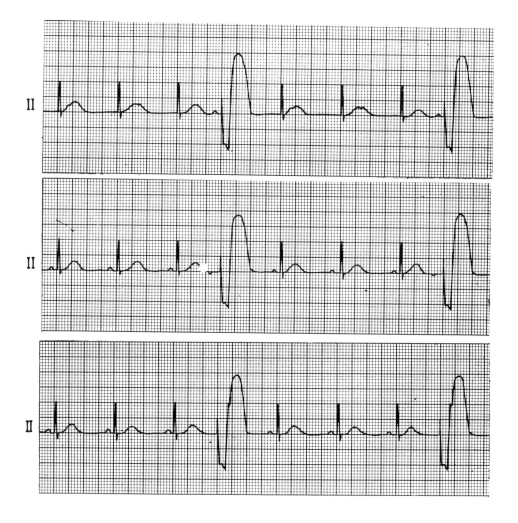

BASIC R-R INTERVAL
REGULAR, BUT INTERRUPTED
INTERMITTENTLY

IRREGULAR R-R INTERVAL
SHORT (PREMATURE QRS)

QRS DURATION OF EARLY COMPLEX
PROLONGED

II

II

II

BASIC R-R INTERVAL
REGULAR, BUT INTERRUPTED
INTERMITTENTLY

IRREGULAR R-R INTERVAL
LONG (DELAYED QRS)

QRS DURATION OF DELAYED COMPLEX
NORMAL

(See Fig. 47.)

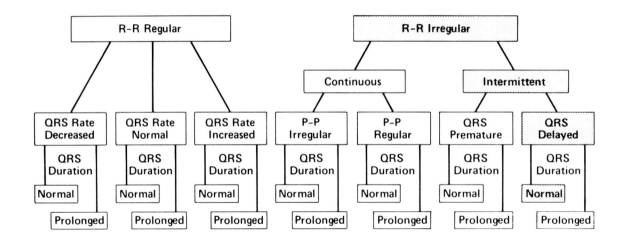

- SUPRAVENTRICULAR RHYTHM WITH INTERMITTENT
  TYPE II SECOND DEGREE AV BLOCK

1. Supraventricular P wave occurs at a regular P-P interval.
2. "Delayed" QRS occurs at twice-preceding R-R interval.
3. "Delayed" QRS is preceded by a supraventricular P wave.

Note. See supraventricular rhythm with fixed type II second degree AV block, page 37.

- SUPRAVENTRICULAR RHYTHM WITH NONCONDUCTED
  PREMATURE ATRIAL CONTRACTION

1. P wave with a different axis or morphology than supraventricular P wave occurs prematurely.
2. "Delayed" QRS complex occurs at less than twice-preceding R-R interval.
3. "Delayed" QRS is preceded by a supraventricular P wave.

Note. See supraventricular rhythm with fixed type II second degree AV block, page 37.

- PAUSE IN SUPRAVENTRICULAR RHYTHM WITH
  ECTOPIC ATRIAL ESCAPE

1. No supraventricular P wave occurs.
2. "Delayed" QRS occurs at more than regular R-R interval.
3. "Delayed" QRS is preceded by a P wave with different axis or morphology than a supraventricular P wave.

- PAUSE IN SUPRAVENTRICULAR RHYTHM WITH
  JUNCTIONAL ESCAPE

1. No supraventricular P wave occurs.
2. "Delayed" QRS occurs at more than regular R-R interval.
3. "Delayed" QRS is not preceded by a P wave.

**BASIC R-R INTERVAL
REGULAR, BUT INTERRUPTED
INTERMITTENTLY**

**IRREGULAR R-R INTERVAL
LONG (DELAYED QRS)**

**QRS DURATION OF DELAYED COMPLEX
NORMAL**

(See Fig. 47.)

BASIC R-R INTERVAL
REGULAR, BUT INTERRUPTED
INTERMITTENTLY

IRREGULAR R-R INTERVAL
LONG (DELAYED QRS)

QRS DURATION OF DELAYED COMPLEX
NORMAL

Figure 47.

Top tracing:

Sinus rhythm with intermittent type II second degree AV block

Basic ventricular and atrial rates = 100/min (R-R and P-P intervals = 0.60 sec). The long R-R interval is 1.20 sec—exactly twice the basic R-R interval—because sinus rhythm continues uninterrupted, despite the blocked P wave.

Second tracing:

Sinus rhythm with nonconducted premature atrial contraction

Basic ventricular and atrial rates = 100/min (R-R and P-P intervals = 0.60 sec). The long R-R interval is 1.0 sec—less than twice the basic R-R interval. The QRS complex preceding the pause is followed by a P wave which occurs at a time when the AV node is refractory and is not conducted to the ventricles. This premature atrial contraction resets the sinus node and sinus rhythm begins again. There is a less than fully compensatory pause following the premature atrial contraction.

Third tracing:

Sinus rhythm with sinus pause and low atrial escape beat

Basic ventricular and atrial rates = 100 min (R-R and P-P interval = 0.60 sec). The long R-R interval is 0.80 sec—longer than the basic R-R interval. The QRS complex preceding the delayed QRS is not followed by a sinus P wave ("pause" in sinus rhythm). The pause is ended by an identical QRS complex which is preceded by a P wave with an axis of 270°–359°—a low atrial escape beat.

Bottom tracing:

Sinus rhythm with sinus pause and junctional escape beat

Basic ventricular and atrial rates = 100/min (R-R and P-P intervals = 0.60 sec). The long R-R interval is 1.0 sec—longer than the basic R-R interval. The pause is longer with a junctional escape beat than with an atrial escape beat because basic junctional rhythm (which determines the escape interval) is slower than atrial rhythm. The QRS complex preceding the delayed QRS is not followed by a sinus P wave ("pause" in sinus rhythm). The pause is ended by an identical QRS complex without a preceding P wave—a junctional escape beat.

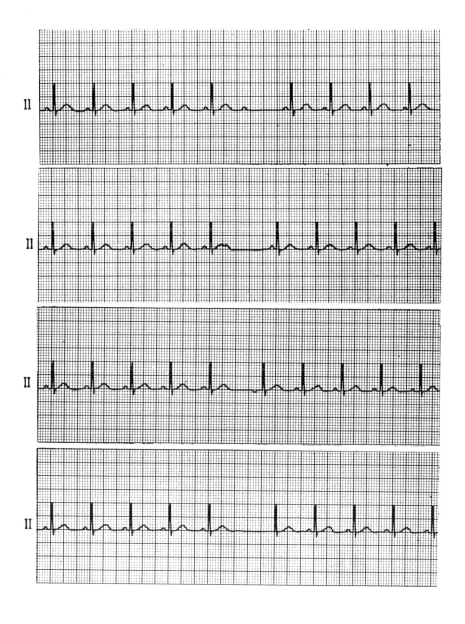

BASIC R-R INTERVAL
REGULAR, BUT INTERRUPTED
INTERMITTENTLY

IRREGULAR R-R INTERVAL
LONG (DELAYED QRS)

QRS DURATION OF DELAYED COMPLEX
NORMAL

BASIC R-R INTERVAL
REGULAR, BUT INTERRUPTED
INTERMITTENTLY

IRREGULAR R-R INTERVAL
LONG (DELAYED QRS)

QRS DURATION OF DELAYED COMPLEX
PROLONGED

(See Fig. 48.)

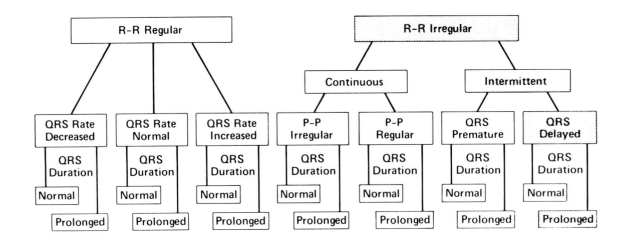

- PAUSE IN SUPRAVENTRICULAR RHYTHM WITH
  VENTRICULAR ESCAPE

1. No supraventricular P wave follows the preceding R wave.
2. "Delayed" QRS occurs at more than regular R-R interval.
3. "Delayed" QRS is not preceded by a P wave.

BASIC R-R INTERVAL
REGULAR, BUT INTERRUPTED
INTERMITTENTLY

IRREGULAR R-R INTERVAL
LONG (DELAYED QRS)

QRS DURATION OF DELAYED COMPLEX
PROLONGED

BASIC R-R INTERVAL
REGULAR, BUT INTERRUPTED
INTERMITTENTLY

IRREGULAR R-R INTERVAL
LONG (DELAYED QRS)

QRS DURATION OF DELAYED COMPLEX
PROLONGED

Figure 48.

Sinus rhythm with sinus pause and ventricular escape beat

Basic ventricular and atrial rates = 100/min (R-R and P-P intervals = 0.60 sec). The long R-R interval is 1.20 sec—longer than the basic R-R interval. The pause is longest with a ventricular escape beat because idioventricular rhythm is the slowest in the heart. The QRS complex preceding the delayed QRS is not followed by a sinus P wave ("pause" in sinus rhythm). The pause is ended by a QRS complex with prolonged duration without a preceding P wave—a ventricular escape beat.

BASIC R-R INTERVAL
REGULAR, BUT INTERRUPTED
INTERMITTENTLY

IRREGULAR R-R INTERVAL
LONG (DELAYED QRS)

QRS DURATION OF DELAYED COMPLEX
PROLONGED

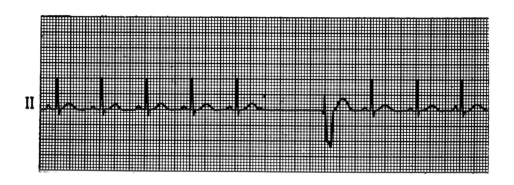

II

Table 1
Electrocardiographic Criteria: Texas Children's Hospital

Normal Values

Age	Heart Rate	Mean Frontal Plane QRS Axis	PR Interval	QRS Duration	Lead V_1 *R Wave Amplitude	Lead V_1 S Wave Amplitude	R/S Ratio	Lead V_6 R Wave Amplitude	Lead V_6 S Wave Amplitude	R/S Ratio
0– 1 mo	100–180 (120)†	+75 to 180 (+120)	.08–.12 (.10)	.04–.08 (.06)	4–25 (15)	0–20 (10)	0.5 to ∞ (1.5)	1–21 (6)	0–12 (4)	0.1 to ∞ (2)
2– 3 mo	110–180 (120)	+35 to +135 (+100)	.08–.12 (.10)	.04–.08 (.06)	2–20 (11)	1–18 (7)	0.3 to 10.0 (1.5)	3–20 (10)	0–6 (2)	1.5 to ∞ (4)
4–12 mo	100–180 (150)	+30 to +135 (+60)	.09–.13 (.12)	.04–.08 (.06)	3–20 (10)	1–16 (8)	0.3 to 4.0 (1.2)	6–20 (13)	0–4 (2)	2.0 to ∞ (6)
1– 3 yr	100–180 (130)	0 to +110 (+60)	.10–.14 (.12)	.04–.08 (.06)	1–18 (9)	1–27 (13)	0.5 to 1.5 (0.8)	3–24 (12)	0–4 (2)	3.0 to ∞ (20)
4– 5 yr	60–150 (100)	0 to +110 (+60)	.11–.15 (.13)	.05–.09 (.07)	1–18 (7)	1–30 (14)	0.1 to 1.5 (0.7)	4–24 (13)	0–4 (1)	2.0 to ∞ (20)
6– 8 yr	60–130 (100)	−15 to +110 (+60)	.12–.16 (.14)	.05–.09 (.07)	1–18 (7)	1–30 (14)	0.1 to 1.5 (0.7)	4–24 (13)	0–4 (1)	2.0 to ∞ (20)
9–11 yr	50–110 (80)	−15 to +110 (+60)	.12–.17 (.14)	.05–.09 (.07)	1–16 (6)	1–26 (16)	0.1 to 1.0 (0.5)	4–24 (14)	0–4 (1)	4.0 to ∞ (20)
12–16 yr	50–100 (75)	−15 to +110 (+60)	.12–.17 (.15)	.05–.09 (.07)	1–16 (5)	1–23 (14)	0 to 1.0 (0.3)	4–22 (14)	0–5 (1)	2.0 to ∞ (9)
>16 yr	50– 90 (70)	−15 to +110 (+60)	.12–.20 (.15)	.05–.10 (.08)	1–14 (3)	1–23 (10)	0 to 1.0 (0.3)	4–21 (10)	0–6 (1)	2.0 to ∞ (9)

SOURCES FOR NORMAL VALUES

Liebman J, Plonsey R. Electrocardiography. In Moss AJ, Adams FH, Emmanouilides GC (eds), Heart Disease in Infants, Children and Adolescents (2nd Ed). Baltimore, Williams & Wilkins, 1977

McCammon RW. A longitudinal study of electrocardiographic intervals in healthy children. Acta Paed Scand 50 (Suppl 126):1–54, 1961

Sreenivasan V, Fisher BJ, Liebman J, Downs TD. Longitudinal study of the standard electrocardiogram in the healthy premature infant during the first year of life. Am J Cardiol 31:57, 1973

Ziegler RF. Electrocardiographic Studies in Normal Infants and Children. Springfield, Ill, Charles C Thomas, 1951

Chamber Enlargement ("Hypertrophy")

Right Ventricular
1. QR pattern in V_{4R}, V_{3R}, or V_1 (may be ventricular inversion)
2. Upright T wave in V_{4R}, V_{3R} or V_1, 5 days-adolescence (may be reciprocal from left chest)
3. Abnormal R/S ratio in V_1 or V_6 (see Table)
4. Abnormal amplitude R wave in V_1 or S wave in V_6

Left Ventricular
1. R wave in V_6 + S wave in V_1 ≥ 60 (Do not use transition leads. Use V_5 if R in V_5 > R in V_6.)
2. S wave in V_1 > 2X R wave in V_5
3. Abnormal R/S ratio
4. Abnormal amplitude R wave in V_1 or R in V_6

Combined Ventricular
1. Meets criteria for RVH *and* S in V_1 or R in V_6 exceeds *mean* for age
2. Meets criteria for LVH *and* R in V_1 or S in V_6 exceeds *mean* for age
3. Equiphasic large midprecordial voltage - weak criterion ("Katz-Wachtel") 65mm in 1 lead, 45mm in 4 leads. (In the presence of complete bundle branch block, criteria for ventricular hypertrophy are invalid.)

Right Atrial
Peaked P wave > 3mm if < 6 months, > 2.5mm ≥ 6 months

Left Atrial
1. Lead II: P wave > 0.09 sec duration
2. Lead V_1: late negative deflection > .04 sec and > 1mm deflection

Combined Atrial
Early portion of P wave peaked (> 2.5mm) *plus* P wave duration > .09 sec.

QT Interval

R-R Interval HR	QT Interval Mean Min–Max	(Mean)
40	1.5 .38–.50	(.45)
50	1.2 .36–.48	(.43)
60	1.0 .34–.46	(.41)
70	0.86 .32–.43	(.37)
80	0.75 .29–.40	(.35)
90	0.67 .27–.37	(.33)
100	0.60 .26–.35	(.30)
120	0.50 .24–.32	(.28)
150	0.40 .21–.28	(.25)
180	0.33 .19–.27	(.23)
200	0.30 .18–.25	(.22)

T Waves

Age	Upright	±	Inverted
0–5 days	I,II,V_6	III,aV_F,V_1	aV_R,V_2–V_5
6 days–2 yrs	I,II,aV_F,V_6	III,V_5	aV_R,V_1–V_4
3 yrs–teens	I,II,aV_F,V_5,V_6	III	aV_R,V_1–V_4
Adults	I,II,III,aV_F,V_1,V_5,V_6	V_2–V_4	aV_R

ST Segment

Elevation or depression > 1mm = myocardial injury.

Elevation without reciprocal depression = injury/pericarditis.

Depression without reciprocal elevation = injury/digitalis/ "normal" premature.

*If QRS duration is normal, add R + R′ and compare total (R + R′) with standards.
∞ R/S undefined because S can be equal to 0.
† Minimum–maximum (mean)

Table 2
Antidysrhythmic Drug Dosages

Drug	Mg/Kg PO		Mg/Kg IV	
Atropine	—		0.01–0.03	
Digoxin: Total digitalizing dose†	0.06		0.04	
maintenance§	0.0075–0.01	q12h	0.004–0.006	q12h
Disopyramide	2.0	q12h	—	
Lidocaine	—		1.0	bolus, then 1 mg/Kg/ hr drip
Phenytoin	2.5–5.0	q12h	10.0–15.0*	
Procainamide	—		10.0–15.0*	
Propranolol	0.5–1.5	q6h	0.01–0.1**	
Quinidine Sulfate	7.5–10.0	q6h	—	

*Give over 1 hour in five divided bolus doses. Watch for hypotension.
**Give only if electrode catheter is in the heart for emergency pacing.
†Maximum total digitalizing dose = 1.0 mg.
§Maximum maintenance dose = 0.125 mg bid.

Sinus Rhythm

CRITERIA

- R-R interval is regular
- QRS rate is normal
- P wave precedes each QRS complex
- P wave axis is 0° to 90° (with normal atrial situs)
- P wave axis remains constant
- PR interval is normal for age and HR
- PR interval remains constant

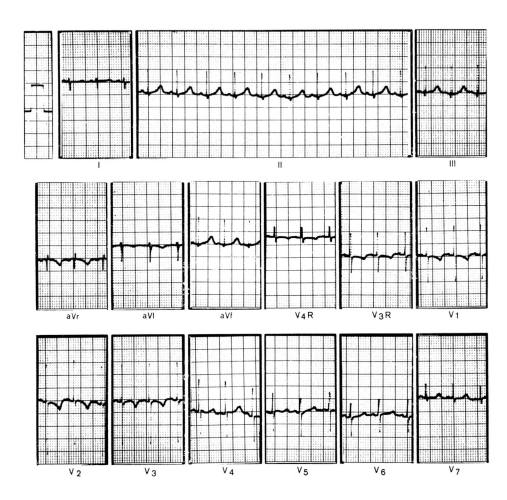

Figure 49.

History: 1-month-old healthy baby

Interpretation: Ventricular and atrial rate 135/min; P axis +30°; PR interval 0.09 sec

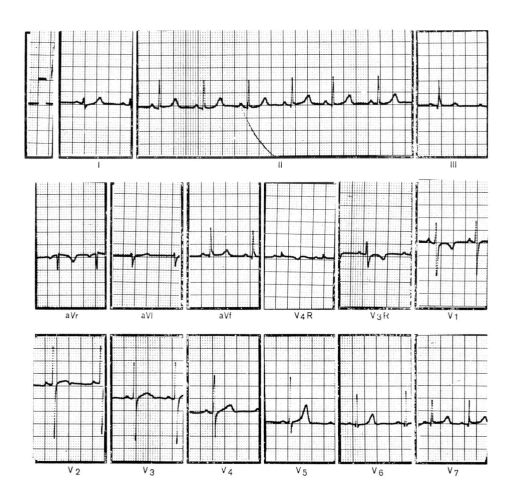

Figure 50.

History: 10-year-old healthy boy

Interpretation: Ventricular and atrial rate 85/min; P axis +60°; PR interval 0.14 sec

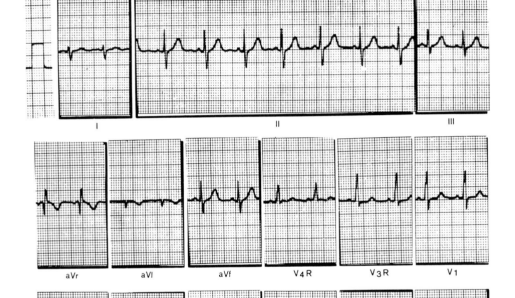

Figure 51.

History: 6-year-old asymptomatic girl with mild pulmonary valve stenosis (preoperative)

Interpretation: Ventricular and atrial rate 90/min; P axis +90°; PR interval 0.12 sec

Additional diagnosis: Right ventricular hypertrophy

Disturbances of Cardiac Rate and Rhythm

Sinus Arrhythmia

CRITERIA

- R-R interval is irregular
- R-R interval varies continuously
- R-R interval is phasic with respiration; increases during inspiration
- "Marked sinus arrhythmia"—variation in rate by 100% (eg, from 50/min to 100/min)
- P-P interval is irregular
- P wave precedes each QRS complex
- P wave axis may vary between 0°–90°
- PR interval varies less than 0.02 sec

CLINICAL SITUATIONS

- Almost always normal
- "Marked sinus arrhythmia"—asthma, airway obstruction, increased intracranial pressure, or may be found in normal children
- Drugs: digitalis or propranolol effect

DIFFERENTIAL DIAGNOSIS

- Premature atrial contraction
- Tachycardia-bradycardia ("sick sinus") syndrome
- Wandering atrial pacemaker

TREATMENT

No specific treatment for sinus arrhythmia if rate is greater than 50/min; if rate is less than 50/min or if symptoms are of low cardiac output, give atropine (see Table 2)

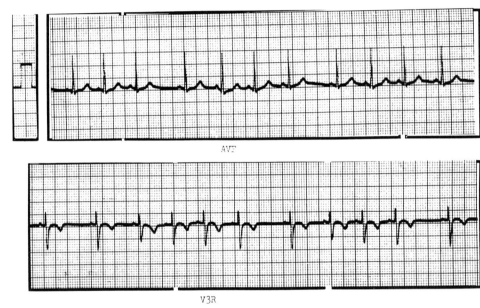

AVF

V3R

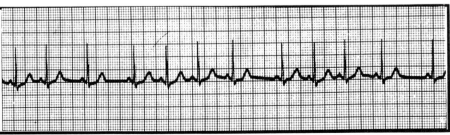

II

Figure 52.

    History: 6-year-old healthy girl

Interpretation: Rate varies from 75/min to 110 min; P axis constant

Wandering Pacemaker

CRITERIA

- R-R interval is irregular
- R-R interval varies continuously
- P-P interval is irregular
- P wave axis continually changes—sinus, atrial, junctional
- QRS complexes are related to all P waves—either P precedes QRS (sinus, atrial origin of P wave) or follows QRS (junctional origin of P wave); P waves may not be visible following junctional beats
- PR interval may vary by up to 0.04 sec

CLINICAL SITUATIONS

- Almost always occurs in otherwise healthy children
- Acute rheumatic fever, asthma, upper airway obstruction
- Rarely results from increased vagal tone (increased intracranial pressure, increased blood pressure, pharyngeal stimulation, abdominal distention)
- Drugs: digitalis or propranolol effect

DIFFERENTIAL DIAGNOSIS

- Premature atrial contraction
- Supraventricular tachycardia
- Tachycardia-bradycardia ("sick sinus") syndrome
- Sinus arrhythmia

TREATMENT

No specific treatment is required if rate is greater than 50/min; if rate is less than 50/min or if symptoms are of low cardiac output, give atropine (see Table 2)

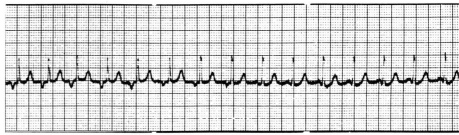

III

III

AVF

Figure 53.

History: 20-month-old healthy girl

Interpretation: P axis continually shifts from positive to negative in leds III and aV$_F$, indicating change in focus from high to low atrial; PR interval remains 0.12 sec despite change in P axis.

Atrial Rhythm

CRITERIA

- R-R interval is regular
- QRS rate is normal
- P wave precedes each QRS complex
- P axis is abnormal
- P axis remains constant
- PR interval may be short; up to 0.04 sec less than normal (see normal values, Table 1)
- PR interval remains constant

CLINICAL SITUATIONS

- May occur in otherwise normal heart
- Increased vagal tone (increased intracranial pressure, increased blood pressure, pharyngeal stimulation, abdominal distention)
- Tachycardia-bradycardia ("sick sinus") syndrome
- Drugs: digitalis

DIFFERENTIAL DIAGNOSIS

- Premature atrial contraction
- Supraventricular tachycardia
- Junctional rhythm

TREATMENT

- No specific treatment is required
- Observe patients with left atrial rhythm closely for episodes of supraventricular tachycardia

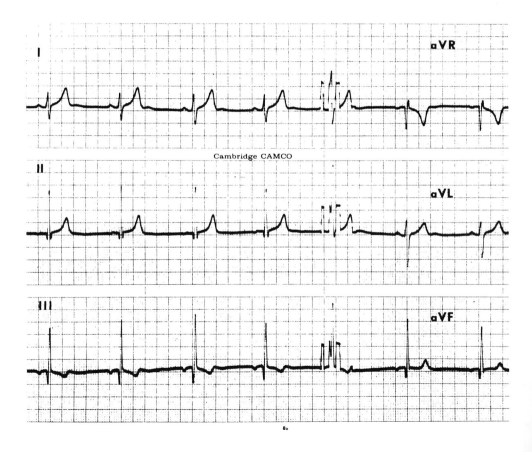

Figure 54.

      History: 16-year-old healthy athletic boy

Interpretation: Ventricular and atrial rate 48/min; P axis −90°; PR interval 0.18 sec

Additional diagnosis: Atrial bradycardia

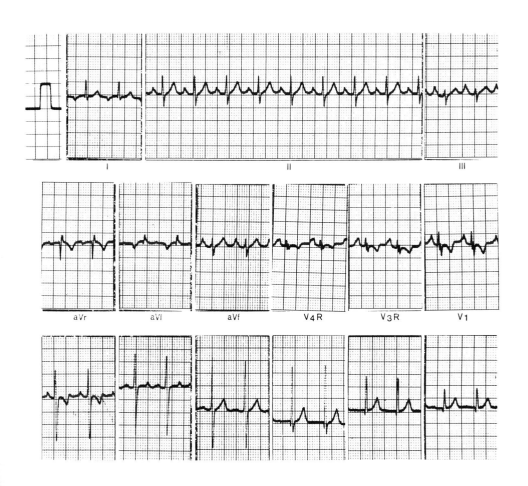

Figure 55.

History: 5-year-old asymptomatic boy

Interpretation: Ventricular and atrial rate 120/min; P morphology in lead V_1 has been called "dome and dart," indicative of left atrial pacemaker; P axis $+120°$; PR interval 0.17 sec

Additional diagnosis: First degree AV block

Sinus Bradycardia

CRITERIA

- R-R interval is regular
- QRS rate is decreased (see normal values, Table 1)
- P wave precedes each QRS complex
- P wave axis is 0°–90° (with normal atrial situs)
- P wave axis remains constant
- PR interval is normal for child's age
- PR interval remains constant

CLINICAL SITUATIONS

- Associated with apnea in "healthy" premature babies
- Increased vagal tone (increased intracranial pressure, increased blood pressure, pharyngeal stimulation, abdominal distention)
- Trained athletes
- Acute rheumatic fever, hypothermia
- Eletrolyte abnormality, hypoxia, hypoglycemia
- Surgery: following any open heart procedure
- Drugs: digitalis or propranolol effect

DIFFERENTIAL DIAGNOSIS

- Second degree AV block, third degree AV block
- Junctional rhythm
- Blocked premature atrial contraction

TREATMENT

- Treat cause
- Atropine for acute treatment of symptomatic bradycardia (see Table 2)

MONITOR LEAD II

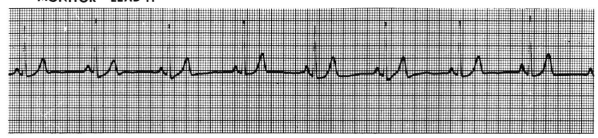

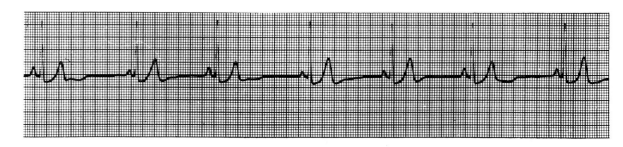

Figure 56.

History: 14-year-old healthy athlete; tracings taken while patient was asleep

Interpretation: Ventricular and atrial rate 42/min

Additional diagnosis: Sinus arrhythmia

Sinus Tachycardia

CRITERIA

- R-R interval is regular
- QRS rate is increased (see normal values, Table 1)
- QRS rate $\leq$ 230/min
- P wave precedes each QRS complex
- P wave axis is 0°–90° (with normal atrial situs)
- P wave axis remains constant
- PR interval is normal for child's age
- PR interval remains constant

CLINICAL SITUATIONS

- Any condition requiring increased cardiac output (thyrotoxicosis, postprandial, exercise, fever, infection, anemia, anxiety, hypovolemia)
- Congestive heart failure
- Myocarditis, acute rheumatic fever
- Drugs: decongestants, isoproterenol

DIFFERENTIAL DIAGNOSIS

- Supraventricular tachycardia;
  usually sinus tachycardia has:
    1. visible P waves
    2. gradual onset in response to clinical situation
    3. gradual slowing in response to the vagal maneuvers of carotid sinus stimulation or Valsalva

TREATMENT

- Treat cause
- Primary treatment to slow rate is not indicated

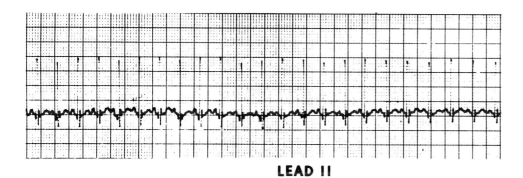

LEAD II

Figure 57.

History: 3-week-old infant with bacterial septicemia

Interpretation: QRS and P rate 220/min

127

Figure 58.

History: 10-year-old healthy boy, one year following repair of tetralogy of Fallot; tracing taken from 24-hour ambulatory
monitor
>   tracing a.—during exercise
>   tracing b.—after exercise
>   tracing c.—at rest

Interpretation:
>   tracing a.—P waves not discernible at beginning
>   with rate 160/min
>   tracing b.—P waves visible at end with rate 150/min
>   tracing c.—sinus rhythm

Additional diagnosis: CRBBB

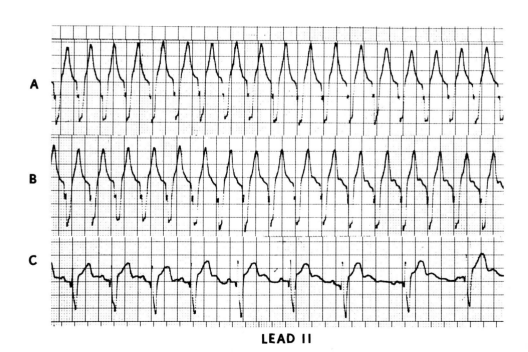

LEAD II

Premature Atrial Contractions

CRITERIA
- Basic R-R interval is regular, but interrupted intermittently
- Irregular R-R interval is short (premature QRS)
- QRS duration of early complex is usually normal; the QRS duration may be prolonged; as long as the other criteria are met and the QRS duration is prolonged, this is a premature atrial contraction with aberration
- P wave precedes each QRS complex

Note. A "nonconducted premature atrial contraction" has an entirely different appearance. The P wave occurs so early in the cycle (usually on the T wave of the preceding QRS complex) that the atrial depolarization fails to conduct to the ventricles and cause a QRS complex, but the premature atrial depolarization is able to discharge the sinus node. Therefore, on the surface ECG the appearance is of a premature P wave and a delayed QRS. (See Figure 18.)

- P axis or morpholgy is usually different from a regular P wave

CLINICAL SITUATIONS
- Usually otherwise normal heart
- Atrial enlargement
- Mechanical (central venous pressure catheter)
- Electrolyte abnormality, hypo..ia, hypoglycemia
- Drugs: digitalis, sympathomimetic amines
- Surgery: following any atrial surgery (rare)

DIFFERENTIAL DIAGNOSIS
- Premature ventricular contraction; premature junctional contraction
- Wandering atrial pacemaker
- Sinus arrhythmia

TREATMENT
- Usually none required (treat cause, if possible)
- Premature atrial contractions which require treatment (digitalis $\pm$ propranolol; see Table 2):
    1. associated with low cardiac output
    2. associated with supraventricular tachycardia or atrial flutter
    3. symptomatic palpitations

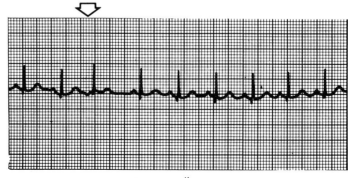

II

Figure 59.

History: 3-year-old boy referred for an irregular heart rate; no treatment was given

Interpretation: Arrow marks premature P wave with a different axis from sinus P waves

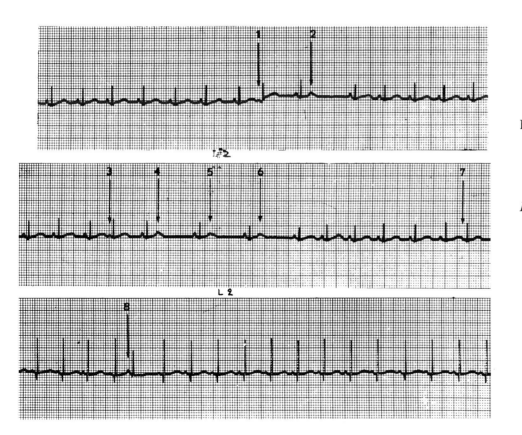

Figure 60.

History: Healthy 2-day-old infant; premature atrial contractions disappeared in 48 hours

Interpretation: Basic R-R and P-P interval 0.50 sec (ventricular and atrial rate 120/min)

Arrows 1, 3, 7—premature atrial contractions with P-P interval 0.40 sec conducted to ventricles without QRS aberration

Arrow 8—premature atrial contraction with P-P interval 0.30 conducted to ventricles with QRS aberration

Arrows 2, 4, 5, 6—premature atrial contractions (P wave on T wave) with P-P interval 0.25—not conducted to ventricles

Supraventricular Tachycardia

CRITERIA

- R-R interval is usually regular (may be irregular in the presence of AV block)
- QRS rate is usually increased (may be normal or decreased in the presence of AV block)
- QRS duration is usually normal (>90 percent)
- P waves
  - most commonly are not visible
  - less commonly follow each QRS with a short R-P interval and inverted P wave in leads II, III, and aV_F ("retrograde" P wave)
  - less commonly precede each QRS with a normal PR interval
  - least commonly are unrelated to QRS (AV dissociation)
- Sudden onset and sudden termination

CLINICAL SITUATIONS

- Otherwise normal heart
- Structural congenital heart disease
- Wolff-Parkinson-White syndrome
- Sepsis, myocarditis, hyperthyroidism, increased intracranial pressure (all rare)
- Drugs (sympathomimetics)
- Surgery: following any type of cardiac surgery

DIFFERENTIAL DIAGNOSIS

- Ventricular tachycardia
- Sinus tachycardia

TREATMENT

Acute Rx (see Table 2)
    Vagal stimulation maneuvers (rarely effective in small children)
    DC electrical cardioversion (synchronized)
    Overdrive atrial pacing with electrode catheter
    Phenylephrine
    Digitalis
Chronic Rx (see Table 2)
    Digitalis
    Propranolol
    Quinidine

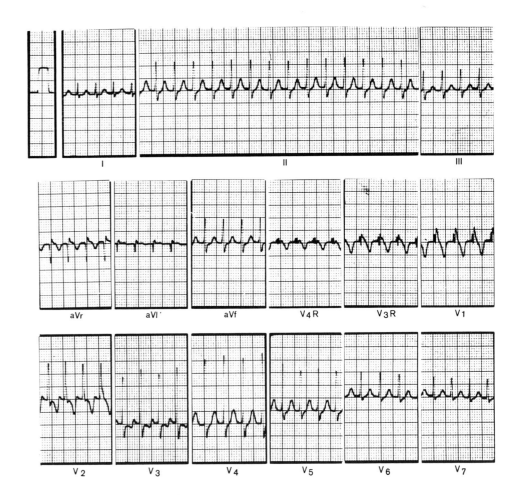

Figure 61.

History: 5-year-old boy with secundum atrial septal defect. After DC electrical cardioversion, ECG showed Wolff-Parkinson-White; chronic treatment was successful with digitalis and quinidine

Interpretation: Ventricular rate 220/min; P waves not visible

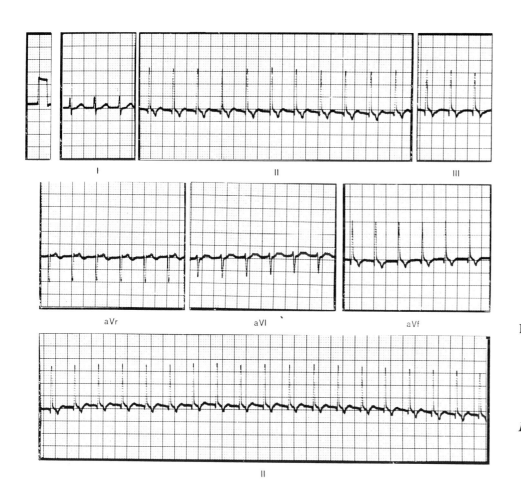

Figure 62.

History: 7-year-old girl with increased intracranial pressure following automobile accident; sinus rhythm resulted after cranial decompression

Interpretation: Ventricular rate 150/min; P waves visible and inverted in leads II, III, aV$_F$ ("retrograde" P waves); PR interval 0.30 sec

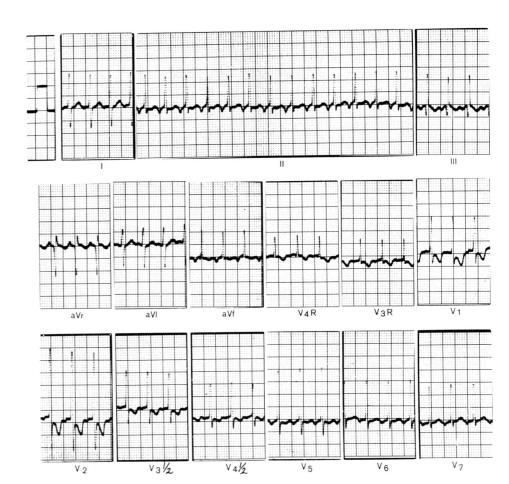

Figure 63.

History: 2-year-old girl with otherwise normal heart; cardioversion failed to convert rhythm; digitalis and propranolol treatment resulted in sinus rhythm

Interpretation: Ventricular rate 180/min; P waves visible and inverted in leads II, III, aV$_F$; PR interval 0.12 sec

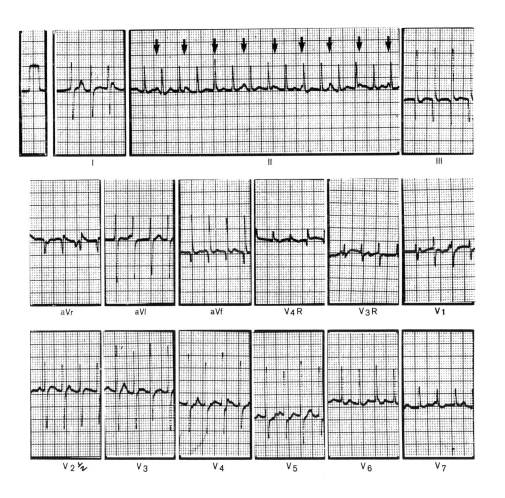

Figure 64.

History: 20-month-old boy suddenly developed this rhythm after trans-atrial repair of a ventricular septal defect. DC electrical cardioversion and overdrive atrial pacing were unsuccessful; intravenous propranolol resulted in marked sinus bradycardia necessitating initiation of atrial pacing. The tachycardia returned at a slower rate and was controlled with propranolol.

Interpretation: Junctional rate 225/min, sinus rate 125/min; the P waves (arrows in lead II) are antegrade from sinus; the QRS complexes originate from a junctional focus and are unrelated to the P waves (AV dissociation).

137

Atrial Flutter

CRITERIA

- R-R interval is usually regular (may be irregular in the presence of AV block)
- QRS rate is usually increased (may be normal or decreased in the presence of AV block)
- Atrial impulses transmit to ventricle with 1 : 1 conduction—ventricular rate usually 300/min; 2 : 1 conduction—ventricular rate usually 150/min; 3 : 1 conduction—ventricular rate 75–150/min
- "Sawtooth" configuration of flutter waves
- Atrial rate is 250–500/min (usually 300/min)

CLINICAL SITUATIONS

- Right or left atrial enlargement
- Tachycardia-bradycardia ("sick sinus") syndrome
- Electrolyte abnormality, hypoxia, hypoglycemia
- Following any atrial surgery

DIFFERENTIAL DIAGNOSIS

- Sinus tachycardia
- Supraventricular tachycardia
- Atrial fibrillation

TREATMENT

Acute Rx (see Table 2)
    DC electrical cardioversion
    Overdrive atrial pacing with electrode catheter
    IV digoxin
    If digitalized, IV procainamide
Chronic Rx (see Table 2)
    If patient still has atrial flutter while receiving digoxin, propranolol or quinidine may be added

Note. Propranolol and quinidine are contraindicated in sick sinus syndrome.

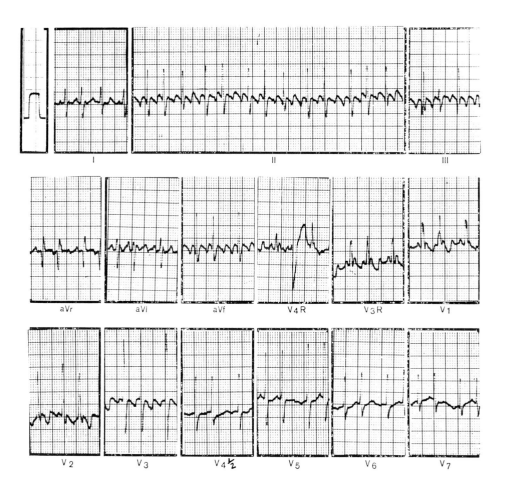

Figure 65.

History: 3-month-old infant with transposition of the great arteries who had balloon atrial septostomy at 3 days of age. DC electrical cardioversion was successful in converting the atrial flutter to sinus rhythm; he had no recurrences on chronic digoxin treatment.

Interpretation: Average ventricular rate 180/min; atrial rate 375/min with sawtooth configuration of atrial flutter; there is alternating 2 : 1 and 3 : 1 AV block. The second QRS complex in V_{4R} with CLBBB morphology results from aberrant conduction of atrial flutter ("Ashman phenomenon").

Figure 66.

History: 3-year-old boy, 18 months following Mustard operation for transposition of the great arteries. At this time, he was being treated with high doses of digoxin and propranolol; a ventricular pacemaker was implanted the following day.

Interpretation: Average ventricular rate 30–80/min; atrial rate 300/min with variable AV block 3 : 1 to 10 : 1

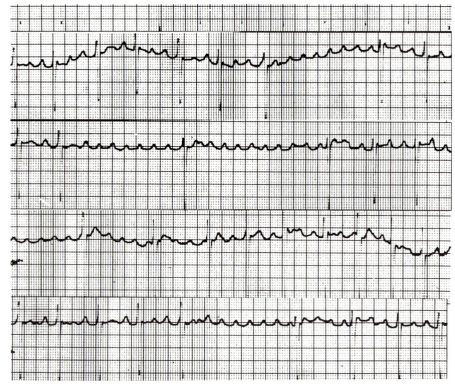

LEAD V$_5$

Atrial Fibrillation

CRITERIA

- R-R interval is irregular
- R-R interval varies continuously (all R-R intervals are usually different)
- Rapid irregular atrial rate with jagged irregular baseline
- Same ECG tracings may have periods of atrial flutter and atrial fibrillation ("atrial flutter-fibrillation")

CLINICAL SITUATIONS

- Rare in children
- Right and left atrial enlargement
- Electrolyte abnormality, hypoxia, hypoglycemia
- Hyperthyroidism
- Following any atrial surgery

DIFFERENTIAL DIAGNOSIS

- Premature atrial contraction
- Premature junctional contraction
- Supraventricular tachycardia
- Atrial flutter

TREATMENT

Acute Rx (see Table 2)
    DC electrical cardioversion
    IV digoxin
Chronic Rx (see Table 2)
    Digitalis
    If patient still has atrial fibrillation while receiving digitalis, then add propranolol or quinidine

Note. Propranolol and quinidine are contraindicated in sick sinus syndrome.

Figure 67.

History: 15-year-old asymptomatic girl with chronic rheumatic mitral regurgitation being treated with digitalis

Interpretation: Simultaneous leads I, II, and III indicate an irregularly-irregular ventricular rate and irregular atrial rate with jagged baseline

Arrow: Brief period of atrial flutter

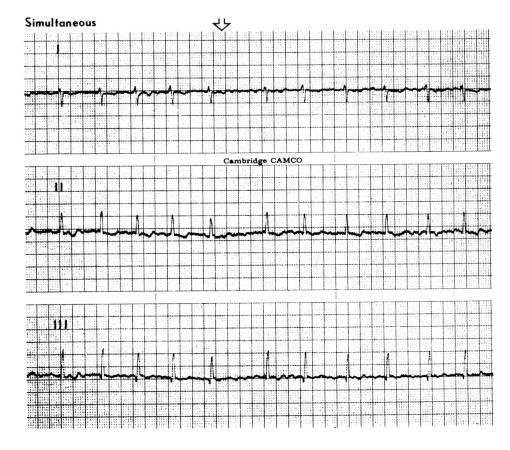

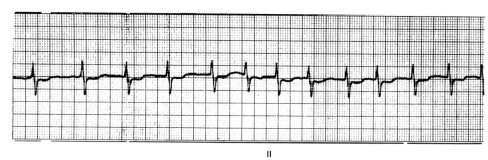

II

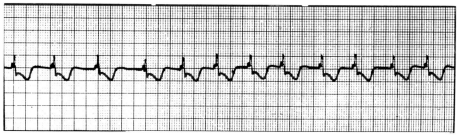

VI

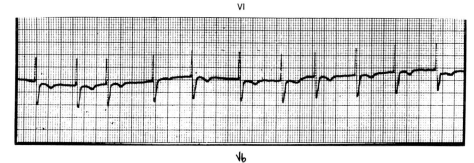

V6

Figure 68.

History: 15-year-old girl with complex cyanotic congenital heart disease and left AV valve regurgitation. She occasionally complained of palpitations and was receiving digitalis.

Interpretation: Ventricular rate is irregularly irregular; baseline is irregular

Premature Junctional Contractions

CRITERIA

- Basic R-R interval is regular, but interrupted intermittently
- Irregular R-R interval is short (premature QRS)
- QRS duration of early complex is normal
- QRS morphology of early complex is similar to regular QRS
- Early QRS is not preceded by a P wave
- If QRS morphology of the early complex is not similar to the regular QRS and there is no preceding P wave, the diagnosis is premature ventricular contraction

CLINICAL SITUATIONS

- Usually otherwise normal heart
- Electrolyte abnormality, hypoxia, hypoglycemia
- Following surgery near AV junction
- Drugs: digitalis toxicity

DIFFERENTIAL DIAGNOSIS

- Premature atrial contraction
- Premature ventricular contraction
- Wandering atrial pacemaker

TREATMENT

- Usually no treatment is required (treat cause if possible)
- Treat with digitalis or propranolol or procainamide (Table 2) if there are signs of low cardiac output, premature junctional contractions are associated with supraventricular tachycardia, or there are symptomatic palpitations

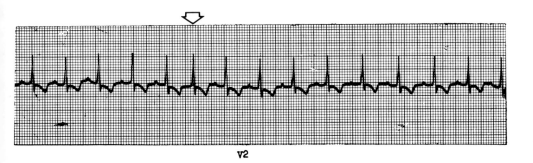

v2

Figure 69.

History: 1-year-old asymptomatic girl with secundum atrial septal defect (preoperative)

Interpretation: Arrow indicates premature QRS complex without a preceding P wave

Junctional Rhythm

CRITERIA

- R-R interval is regular
- QRS rate is decreased (rate of junctional rhythm is 50–90/min in infants and 50–70/min in children)
- QRS duration is normal
- Sinus P rate is less than the QRS rate with AV dissociation; or "retrograde" P wave (axis 270° to 359°) follows some or all QRS complexes with R-P interval < 0.30 sec
- Alternation between sinus rhythm and junctional rhythm is common

CLINICAL SITUATIONS

- Otherwise normal heart
- Tachycardia-bradycardia ("sick sinus") syndrome
- Increased vagal tone (increased intracranial pressure, increased blood pressure, abdominal distention, pharyngeal stimulation)
- Electrolyte abnormality, hypoxia, hypoglycemia
- Following atrial surgery or any open heart surgery

DIFFERENTIAL DIAGNOSIS

- Complete AV block
- Supraventricular tachycardia
- Premature atrial contraction

TREATMENT

- If the ventricular rate is adequate, primary treatment is not indicated
- If symptomatic, treat with atropine or atrial pacing with electrode catheter

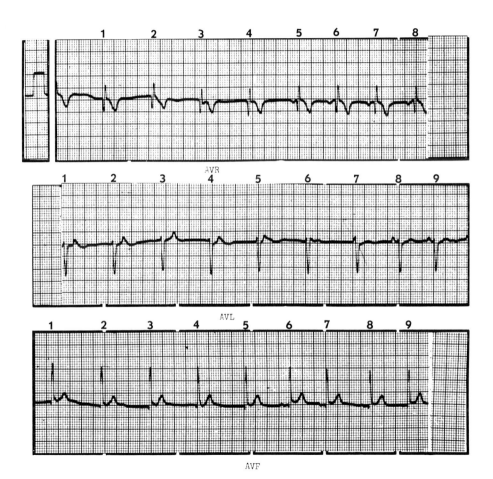

AVR

AVL

AVF

Figure 70.

History: 4-year-old boy, two years after Mustard operation for transposition of the great arteries

Interpretation:

aV_R: first four complexes are junctional at rate 72, then last four are sinus at rate 92 (normal sinus P waves negative in aV_R)

aV_L: first seven complexes are junctional with retrograde P waves visible in first five (note difference in T waves from sinus T waves in last two complexes); retrograde P waves may be upright in aV_L

aV_F: first five complexes junctional with retrograde P waves

147

Accelerated Junctional Rhythm

CRITERIA

- R-R interval is usually regular or intermittently irregular with sinus "capture" beats
- QRS rate is moderately elevated (> 90/min in infants or > 70/min in children), but < 160/min
- Sinus P rate is less than the QRS rate, with AV dissociation; or "retrograde" P wave (axis 270° to 359°) following some or all QRS complexes with R-P interval < 0.30 sec

Note. Accelerated junctional rhythm (or "nonparoxysmal" junctional tachycardia) is a type of "slow" supraventricular tachycardia with either retrograde P waves or AV dissociation. If the ventricular rate is less than 130/min, the rhythm is classified as accelerated junctional rhythm; if the rate is 160/min or more, it is supraventricular tachycardia; if the rate is 130–150/min, it may be classified as either supraventricular tachycardia or accelerated junctional rhythm.

CLINICAL SITUATIONS

- Myocarditis, increased intracranial pressure—rare
- Electrolyte abnormality, hypoxia, hypoglycemia
- Long after any type of cardiac surgery (part of "sick sinus syndrome") or immediately after cardiac surgery near the AV junction
- Drugs: digitalis intoxication, phenytoin intoxication

DIFFERENTIAL DIAGNOSIS

- Supraventricular tachycardia
- Junctional rhythm
- Second degree AV block
- Third degree AV block

TREATMENT

This is usually well tolerated and extremely resistant to treatment (treat cause, if possible)

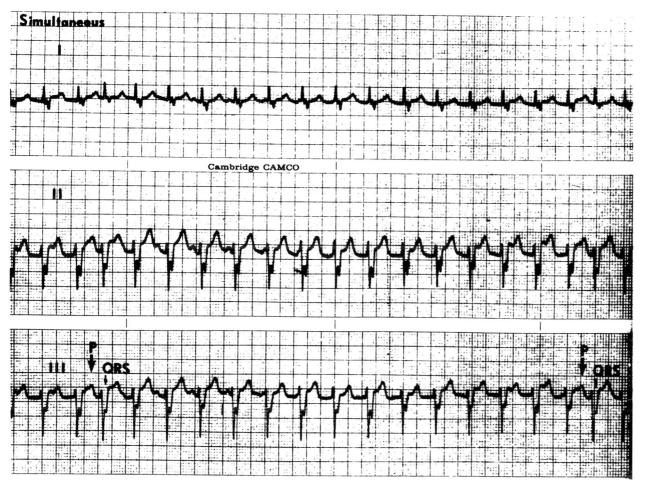

Simultaneous

I

Cambridge CAMCO

II

III

P QRS

P QRS

Figure 71.

History:
7-year-old asymptomatic girl three days following repair of persistent AV canal; no treatment was instituted; stable sinus rhythm occurred 24 hours later.

Interpretation:
Basic R-R interval is regular with QRS rate of 130/min; the P waves are antegrade from the sinus; the QRS complexes are unrelated to the P waves and originate from a junctional focus (AV dissociation). There are two exceptions where the R-R interval is short. In these instances (marked "P" and "QRS"), the sinus impulse is conducted to the ventricles.

Additional diagnosis:
CRBBB with left axis deviation

Premature Ventricular Contractions

CRITERIA

- Basic R-R interval is regular, but interrupted intermittently
- Irregular R-R interval is short (premature QRS)
- QRS duration of premature complex is prolonged
- QRS morphology is different from regular QRS
- "Fusion" complexes—premature ventricular contractions occurring late in diastole depolarize the ventricles simultaneously with the depolarization originating from the sinus node; the resultant QRS complex has a morphology with characteristics of both sinus QRS and PVC
- Premature QRS complex is not preceded by a P wave

CLINICAL SITUATIONS

- Otherwise normal heart
- Mechanical (catheters or pacing wires)
- Electrolyte abnormality, hypoxia, hypoglycemia
- Structural congenital heart disease; cardiomyopathy
- Myocarditis
- Following any cardiac surgery
- Drugs: isoproterenol, digitalis, imipramine

DIFFERENTIAL DIAGNOSIS

- Premature atrial contraction with aberration
- Premature junctional contraction with aberration

TREATMENT

- If the heart is normal and premature ventricular contractions are uniform (same morphology in a single ECG lead) and disappear with exercise, no treatment is needed.
- If the heart is abnormal, or premature ventricular contractions are multiform or do not disappear with exercise:
    Acute Rx: Lidocaine, procainamide (Table 2)
    Chronic Rx: Phenytoin, propranolol, quinidine (Table 2)

Simultaneous

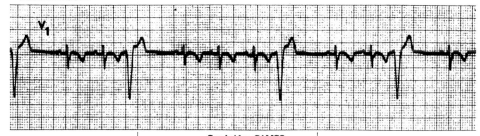

Cambridge CAMCO

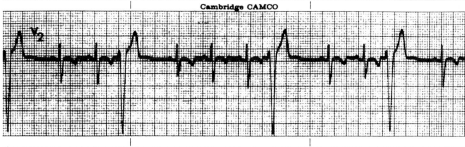

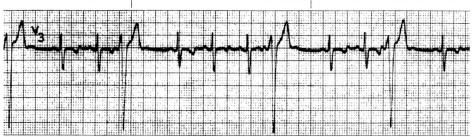

Figure 72.

History: 8-year-old healthy boy in whom physician heard irregular heart rate; ECG normalized during exercise; no treatment was given.

Interpretation: Frequent uniform premature ventricular contractions

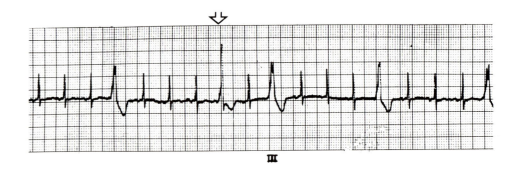

III

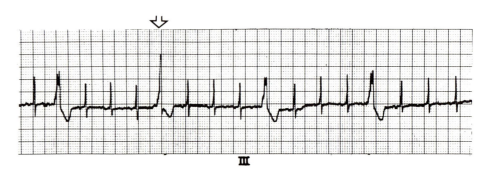

III

Figure 73.

History: 6-month-old healthy infant; no treatment was given

Interpretation: Uniform premature ventricular contractions; arrows mark fusion complexes

Figure 74.

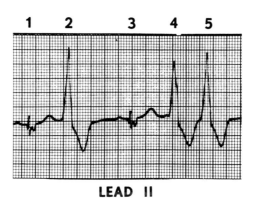

LEAD II

History: 14-year-old, seven years after repair of tetralogy of Fallot; treatment with phenytoin abolished the premature ventricular contractions

Interpretation: Complex 2—single premature ventricular contraction; complexes 4, 5—paired premature ventricular contractions (also called a "couplet")

Additional diagnosis: First degree AV block and CRBBB

Figure 75.

History: 2-year-old girl referred for syncopal episodes; treatment with propranolol was effective at abolishing episodes which were due to ventricular dysrhythmias

Interpretation:
    (a) tracing: "ventricular bigeminy"—alternating sinus beats with premature ventricular contractions
    (b) tracing: couplet (arrow) and bigeminy

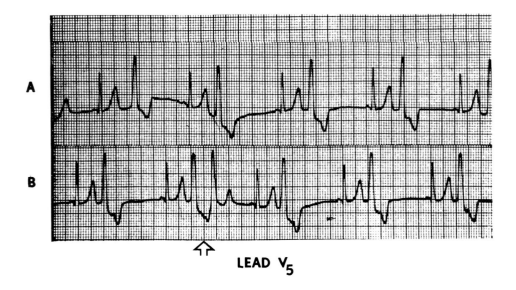

LEAD V$_5$

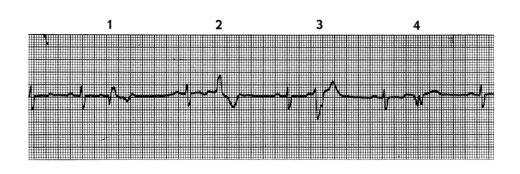

Figure 76.

History: 14-year-old boy, four years after repair of double outlet right ventricle and pulmonary stenosis; despite treatment with digoxin and quinidine, the patient died suddenly

Interpretation: "Multiform" (different morphology in a single ECG lead) premature ventricular contractions; note each complex (labeled 1–4) is a different shape and none is a fusion complex

Ventricular Tachycardia

CRITERIA

- R-R interval is usually regular
- QRS rate is increased ($> 120/\text{min}$)
- QRS duration is prolonged
- QRS morphology is different from regular QRS
- Ventricular origin of tachycardia is substantiated by: fusion beats (in order to have fusion the depolarization must originate from the ventricle); QRS morphology during tachycardia similar to single premature ventricular contractions recorded during predominant sinus rhythm
- P waves: P wave is visible following some or all QRS complexes with constant R-P interval; or no P wave is visible; or sinus P rate is less than QRS rate with AV dissociation
- If the above criteria are met, ventricular tachycardia is defined as three or more beats in a row
- "Slow ventricular tachycardia" or "accelerated ventricular rhythm" meet the above criteria, but have QRS rates of 120/min or less

CLINICAL SITUATIONS

- Otherwise normal heart (rare)
- Prolonged QT interval syndromes (familial—with or without deafness)
- Mechanical (catheters, pacing wires)
- Electrolyte abnormality, hypoxia, hypoglycemia
- Structural congenital heart disease
- Myocarditis, cardiomyopathy
- Following any cardiac surgery
- Drugs: isoproterenol, digitalis, imipramine

DIFFERENTIAL DIAGNOSIS

- Supraventricular tachycardia with aberration

TREATMENT

Acute Rx (Table 2)	Chronic Rx (Table 2)
Electrical DC cardioversion (synchronized)	Propranolol
Lidocaine	Phenytoin
Procainamide	Quinidine

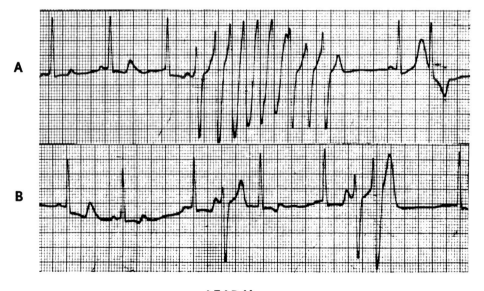

A

B

LEAD II

Figure 77.

History: 6-year-old previously well boy referred after sudden loss of consciousness; propranolol treatment eliminated further episodes of loss of consciousness. His hearing was normal.

Interpretation:

Ventricular tachycardia

Tracing (A): ventricular rate 300/min with morphology similar to single premature ventricular contractions found in tracing (B); the QT interval is prolonged in all sinus complexes.

Figure 78.

History: 17-year-old asymptomatic girl with complex cyanotic congenital heart disease. Propranolol eliminated the ventricular tachycardia, but congestive heart failure resulted. Quinidine treatment was successful.

Interpretation:

Ventricular tachycardia

Tracings (A) and (B): Ventricular rate 125–145; arrows indicate sinus P waves (notches on T waves) continuing through ventricular tachycardia—evidence of AV dissociation

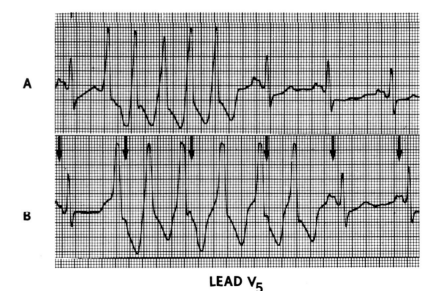

LEAD V$_5$

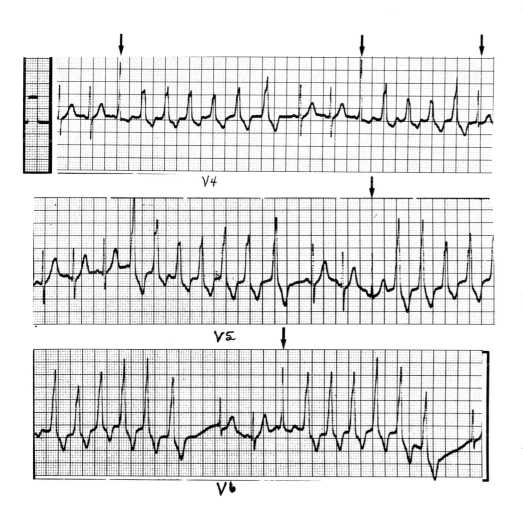

Figure 79.

History: 6-year-old boy, asymptomatic, referred for an irregular heart rate. He had an anatomically normal heart. Treatment with phenytoin and with quinidine did not affect the tachycardia. Combination of the two drugs resulted in fewer episodes, but the tachycardia persisted.

Interpretation: Ventricular tachycardia leads V_4, V_5, V_6; ventricular rate 150/min, sinus rate 125/min; arrows indicate fusion complexes

Disturbances of Cardiac Conduction

First Degree AV Block

CRITERIA

- May occur with any supraventricular rhythm and is due to prolonged conduction from atria to ventricles
- PR interval is prolonged (see normal values, Table 1)

CLINICAL SITUATIONS

- Increased vagal tone (increased intracranial pressure, increased blood pressure, pharyngeal stimulation, gastric distention)
- Myocarditis, acute rheumatic fever
- Structural congenital heart disease
- Following any intracardiac surgery
- Drugs: digitalis, propranolol (first degree AV block is *not* a sign of digitalis or propranolol toxicity, but rather an *effect* of the drug)

DIFFERENTIAL DIAGNOSIS

- AV dissociation
- Second degree AV block
- Third degree AV block

TREATMENT

None necessary

FIRST DEGREE AV BLOCK

Figure 80.

History: 12-year-old girl, six years after repair of primum atrial septal defect

Interpretation: PR interval 0.25 secs; the QT interval is also prolonged

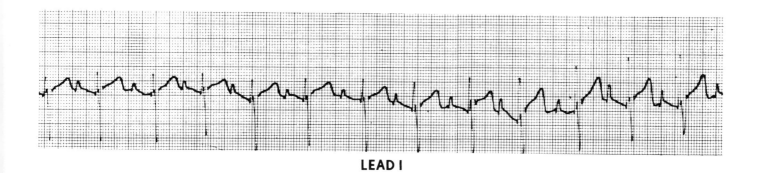

LEAD I

Second Degree AV Block

CRITERIA

- May occur with any supraventricular rhythm and is due to intermittent conduction from the atria to the ventricles
- Type I (Wenckebach)
  - R-R interval is irregular
  - R-R interval varies continuously
  - R-R interval progressively shortens, then prolongs for one interval
  - P-P interval is regular
  - PR interval progressively lengthens until a single P wave is not followed by a QRS complex
- Fixed type II
  - R-R interval is regular
  - P-P interval is regular
  - P rate is a multiple of the QRS rate (eg, 2 : 1, 3 : 1, or 4 : 1)
  - There is a fixed relationship of P waves to QRS complexes
- Varying type II
  - R-R interval is irregular
  - R-R interval varies continuously
  - P-P interval is regular
  - R-R interval is a varying multiple of P-P interval (eg, alternating 2 : 1 and 3 : 1)
  - All R waves are preceded by a P wave with the same PR interval
- "High grade" or "Advanced"
  - R-R interval is regular, but interrupted intermittently
  - Irregular R-R interval is short (premature QRS)
  - P-P interval is regular
  - P waves and QRS complexes are basically unrelated (AV dissociation), except each short R-R interval is preceded by a P wave with a PR interval $\leq$ 0.40 sec
  - In "high grade" block the basically regular R-R interval is usually due to junctional rhythm and the short R-R intervals are due to intermittent AV conduction ("sinus capture beats")

CLINICAL SITUATIONS

- May occur in an otherwise normal heart
- Increased vagal tone (increased intracranial pressure, increased blood pressure, pharyngeal stimulation, gastric distention)
- Myocarditis
- Structural congenital heart disease
- Surgery: following surgery near AV junction
- Drugs: digitalis toxicity usually manifested by Wenckebach

DIFFERENTIAL DIAGNOSIS

- Premature atrial contraction
- AV dissociation
- First degree AV block, third degreee AV block

TREATMENT

- Treat cause
- If patient is symptomatic, a ventricular pacemaker should be implanted

Figure 81.

History: 8-month-old boy with nasogastric tube causing irregular heart rate; the abnormality disappeared when the tube was removed.

Interpretation: Beginning at the arrow, R-R intervals shorten. The P-P interval is regular. PR intervals lengthen (0.16, 0.22, 0.24), and then a P wave without a following QRS occurs. This is called 4 : 3 Wenckebach (four P waves, three QRS complexes).

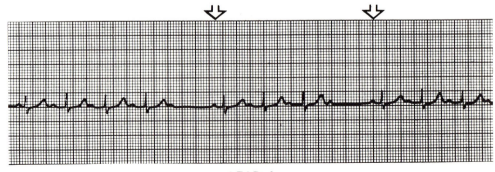

LEAD I

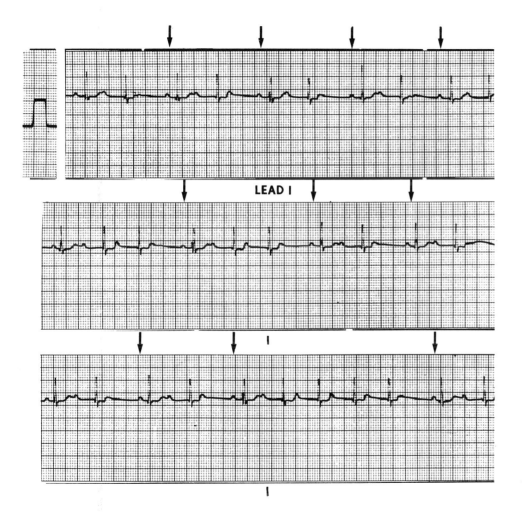

LEAD I

Figure 82.

History: 5-year-old girl, one year following repair of partial anomalous pulmonary venous return. She was receiving no medication; no treatment was given.

Interpretation: Wenckebach sequences begin with each arrow.

169

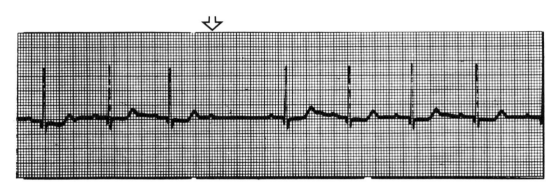

LEAD III

Figure 83.

History: 9-year-old boy who developed irregular heart rate five years after repair of persistent AV canal. Cardiac catheterization determined the block to be below the bundle of His. A permanent pacemaker was implanted.

Interpretation: R-R interval is basically regular, except for a pause exactly twice the basic R-R interval; P-P interval is constant; the PR is constant until a P wave is not followed by a QRS complex.

Figure 84.

History:

15-year-old boy with complex cyanotic congenital heart disease, including ventricular inversion, and a slow, irregular heart rate. Because of increasing symptoms of congestive heart failure, a permanent ventricular pacemaker was implanted.

Interpretation:

The basic rhythm is junctional at 40/min (cycle length 1480 msec); short R-R intervals (complexes 5, 9, and 12) indicate conduction from preceding P waves (arrows).

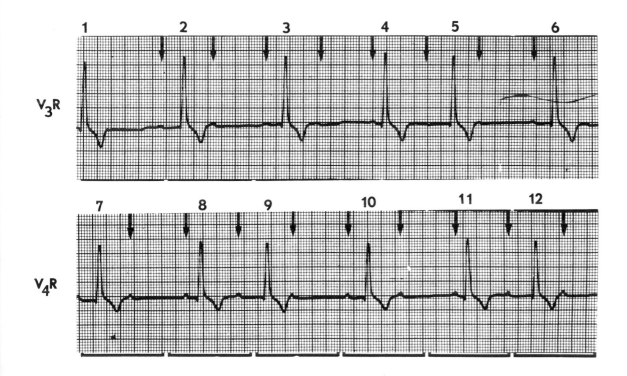

Third Degree (Complete) AV Block

CRITERIA

- May occur with any supraventricular rhythm and is due to complete block in conduction from atria to ventricles
- R-R interval is regular
- QRS rate is decreased
- QRS duration is normal or abnormal
- Complete AV dissociation is present
- The regular R-R interval is usually due to junctional rhythm; if the rhythm originates from below the bundle of His, the QRS duration is prolonged

CLINICAL SITUATIONS

- Congenital—may be associated with ventricular inversion
- Acquired—cardiac surgery, cardiac catheterization
- Myocarditis

DIFFERENTIAL DIAGNOSIS

- First degree AV block
- Second degree AV block
- AV dissociation
- Sinus bradycardia

TREATMENT

Acute Rx
    Atropine
    Isoproterenol
    Temporary ventricular pacing
Chronic Rx
    If low cardiac output, ventricular pacing
    If block is determined to be within or below bundle of His or the patient is symptomatic, ventricular pacing

Figure 85.

History: 11-year-old asymptomatic girl known to have complete AV block resulting from repair of a persistent AV canal. Tracings taken from 24-hour tape ECG performed in routine follow-up; all tracings taken while the patient was asleep. She had immediate pacemaker implantation.

Interpretation: Arrows mark P waves; there is marked sinus arrhythmia.
Tracing A—R-R interval constant at 1.76 sec (heart rate 34/min) with no relationship of P to QRS.
Tracing B—R-R interval lengthens to 1.80 sec between complexes 1–2, and then a 3.12 sec pause occurs before the next QRS complex.
Tracing C—A 7.40 sec pause occurs between QRS complexes. A different focus in the ventricle depolarizes, ending the long pause.

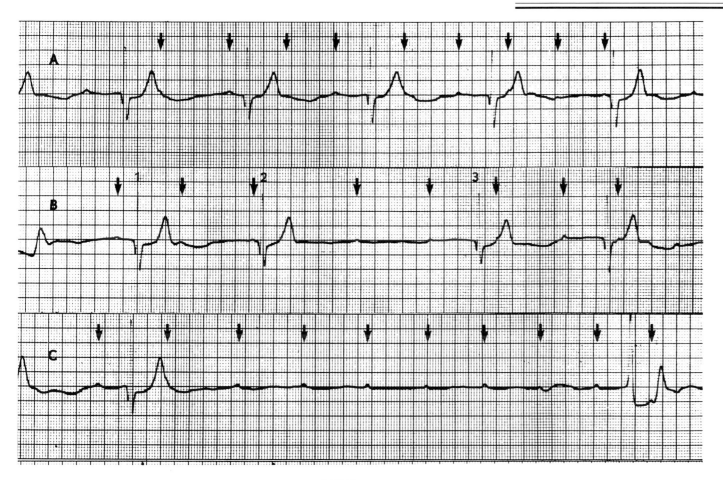

LEAD I

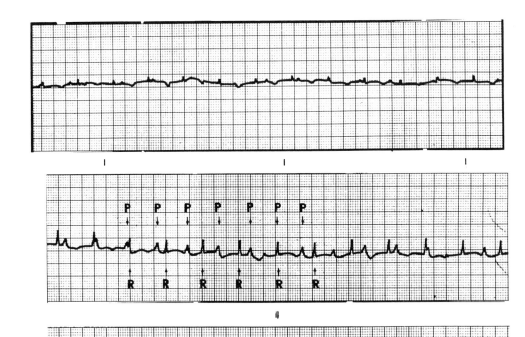

Figure 86.

History: 12-hour-old asymptomatic infant born with slow heart rate; no treatment was required

Interpretation: Ventricular rate 100/min, atrial rate 120/min; no relationship of P waves to QRS complexes; normal QRS duration (0.05 sec)

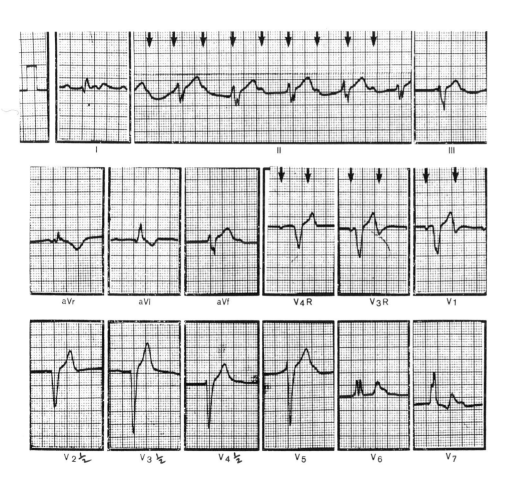

Figure 87.

History: 17-year-old boy developed slow heart rate immediately following aortic valve commissurotomy; cardiac catheterization determined the block to be above the bundle of His; no treatment was given.

Interpretation: Ventricular rate 67/min, atrial rate 130/min. At first glance this appears to be first degree AV block. Arrows indicate P waves; QRS duration is prolonged (0.15 sec) with CLBBB.

Complete Right Bundle Branch Block
(Normal Frontal Plane QRS Axis)

CRITERIA

- Prolonged QRS duration (>0.10 sec in child under 16 years; >0.12 sec over 16 years)
- rsR′ pattern in right chest leads (V_{3R}, V_{4R}, V_1) with initial (0.04 sec) rapid deflection and terminal (0.06–0.08 sec) slow deflection
- Major deflection in leads II, III, aV_F is positive
- No Q wave in leads I, aV_L

CLINICAL SITUATIONS

- Congenital (rare)
- Acquired
  - Related to ventricular rate (can have functional CRBBB with tachycardia or bradycardia—both rare in children)
  - Myocarditis
  - Hypoxia, electrolyte abnormality, hypoglycemia
  - Surgery: most commonly caused by cardiac surgery
  - Drugs: quinidine

DIFFERENTIAL DIAGNOSIS

- Right ventricular hypertrophy (in right ventricular hypertrophy, terminal deflection is rapid)
- Wolff-Parkinson-White

TREATMENT

None

Figure 88.

History: 2-year-old asymptomatic girl, one month after repair of ventricular septal defect; no treatment was given

Interpretation: QRS duration 0.11 sec; rsR′ pattern in right chest leads; major QRS deflection positive in leads II, III, aV_F

Additional diagnosis: First degree AV block

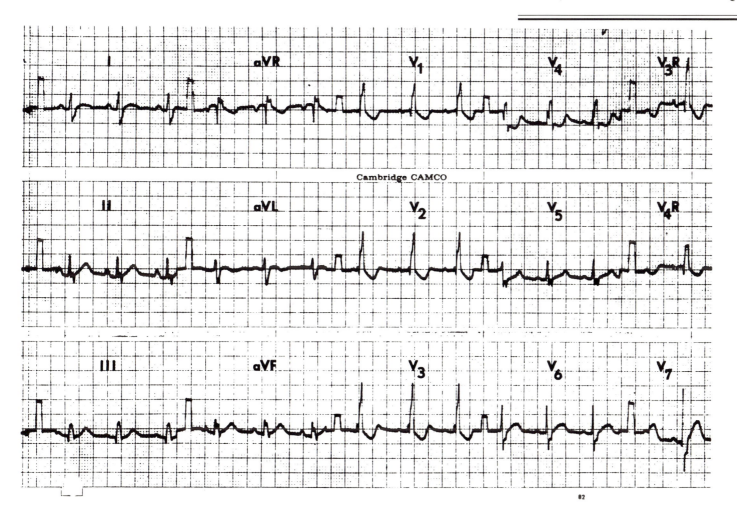

Cambridge CAMCO

COMPLETE RIGHT BUNDLE BRANCH BLOCK WITH
LEFT AXIS DEVIATION

Complete Right Bundle Branch Block with
Left Axis Deviation (Left Anterior Hemiblock)

CRITERIA

- Prolonged QRS duration (>0.10 sec in child under 16 years; >0.12 sec over 16 years)
- rsR' pattern in right chest leads (V_{3R}, V_{4R}, V_1) with initial (0.04 sec) rapid deflection and terminal (0.06–0.08 sec) slow deflection
- Major deflection in leads II, III, aV_F is negative
- Q wave in leads I, aV_L

CLINICAL SITUATIONS

- Congenital (rare)
- Acquired
  - Related to ventricular rate (can have CRBBB with tachycardia or bradycardia—both rare in children)
  - Myocarditis
  - Hypoxia, electrolyte abnormality, hypoglycemia
  - Surgery: most commonly caused by cardiac surgery
  - Drugs: quinidine

DIFFERENTIAL DIAGNOSIS   TREATMENT

- Right ventricular hypertrophy   None

Note. An association has been made between the development of this pattern following cardiac surgery and sudden, unexpected death, presumably from third degree AV block. Whether this association has any cause and effect relationship is controversial. Children who have syncope should undergo intracardiac electrophysiologic study and possible pacemaker implantation.

Figure 89.

History: 12-year-old asymptomatic boy five years following repair of tetralogy of Fallot; no treatment was given.

Interpretation: QRS duration 0.19 sec; rsR' pattern in right chest leads; major QRS deflection negative in leads II, III, aV_F; Q wave leads I, aV_L

Additional diagnosis: First degree AV block

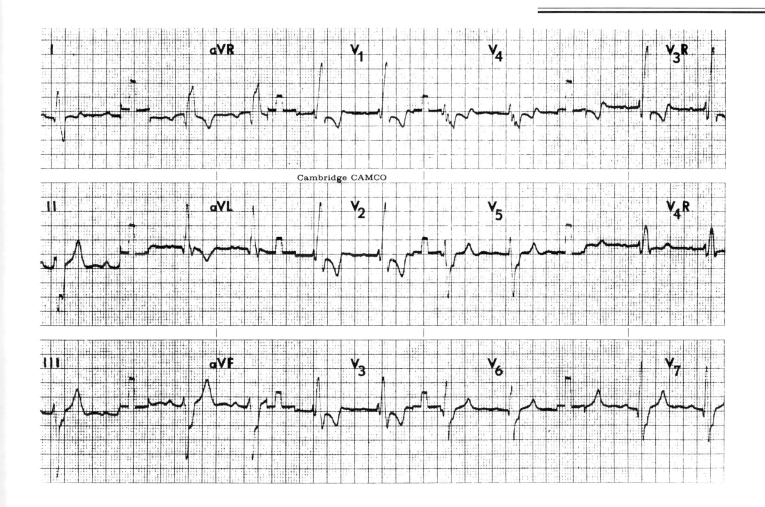

Cambridge CAMCO

Complete Left Bundle Branch Block

CRITERIA

- Prolonged QRS duration (>0.10 sec in a child under 16 years; >0.12 sec over 16 years)
- rR′ morphology (M-shaped) in left chest leads (V_5, V_6) and lead I
- Absent Q wave in left chest leads
- QS pattern in right chest leads

CLINICAL SITUATIONS

- Congenital (rare)
- Acquired
  - Myocarditis
  - Hypoxia, electrolyte abnormality, hypoglycemia
  - Following any cardiac surgery
  - Drugs: quinidine

DIFFERENTIAL DIAGNOSIS

- Left ventricular hypertrophy
- Wolff-Parkinson-White

TREATMENT

None necessary unless associated with syncope or after surgery. Children with CLBBB and syncope or surgical CLBBB should undergo an intracardiac electrophysiologic study and possible pacemaker implantation.

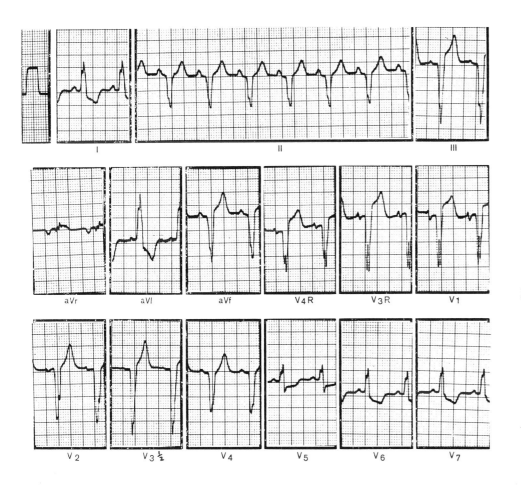

Figure 90.

History: 17-year-old girl was referred for syncope; she had an otherwise normal heart. A ventricular pacemaker was implanted and episodes of syncope (presumably intermittent complete AV block) were abolished.

Interpretation: QRS duration 0.12 sec; rR′ morphology lead I, V_6; absent Q wave lead V_6; qS pattern lead V_1

WOLFF-PARKINSON-WHITE

ACCELERATED CONDUCTION

Wolff-Parkinson-White
CRITERIA

- "Delta wave"—slurred positive or negative initial deflection of QRS complex
- Fusion QRS—early activation of ventricle via Kent bundle gives delta wave; later activation via His bundle gives remainder of QRS
- Short PR (actually P-delta) interval (see normal values for PR, Table 1)
- Not all leads will show a short PR and delta wave (leads with isoelectric delta waves)
- Wolff-Parkinson-White has been separated into type A, B, and C depending on QRS morphology, and this was said to localize the Kent bundle; however, localization of a Kent bundle from the surface ECG is not always possible and we have abandoned this classification.

CLINICAL SITUATIONS

- May be associated with congenital heart disease, especially Ebstein's anomaly and mitral valve prolapse

Note. Wolff-Parkinson-White predisposes to supraventricular tachycardia

DIFFERENTIAL DIAGNOSIS

- Premature atrial contraction
- Premature ventricular contraction
- Sinus tachycardia with Wolff-Parkinson-White may simulate ventricular tachycardia

TREATMENT

None unless supraventricular tachycardia or syncope present (see treatment for supraventricular tachycardia

182

Figure 91.

History: 5-week-old boy with history of rapid heart rate; chronic treatment was successful with digitalis.

Interpretation: P-delta interval (lead V_1) 0.06 sec; positive delta wave leads V_1–V_5; negative delta wave leads II, III, aV_F, V_7

Additional diagnosis: Sinus tachycardia

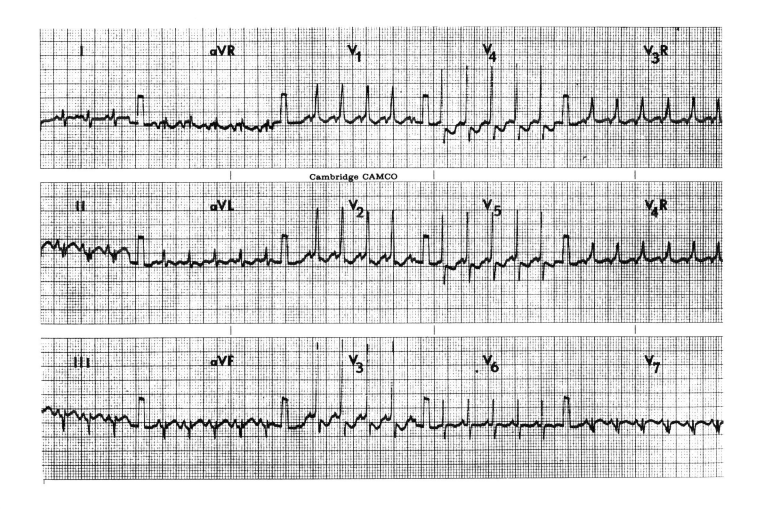

Cambridge CAMCO

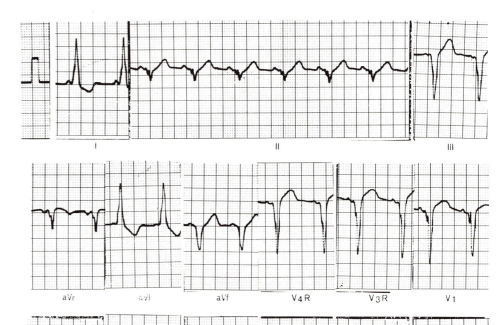

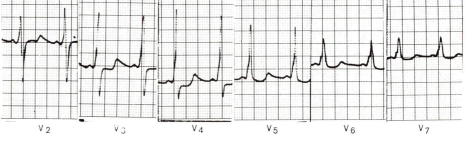

Figure 92.

History: 13-year-old boy admitted to an intensive care unit following reduction of fractured leg; on ECG, found to have short PR interval; he had no history of tachycardia and received no treatment

Interpretation: P-delta interval (lead I) 0.08 sec; left axis deviation of QRS; negative delta wave leads V_{4R}, V_{3R}, V_1; positive delta wave left chest leads

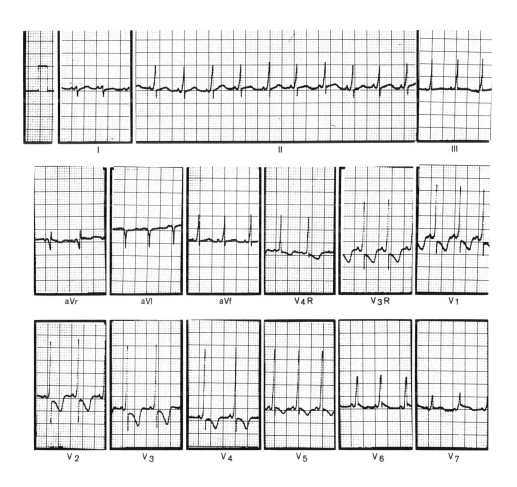

Figure 93.

History: A 15-day-old infant had been born prematurely at 36 weeks gestation. An ECG was obtained as part of an evaluation for cardiac murmur; the murmur was functional; the infant was asymptomatic and so was not treated.

Interpretation: P-delta interval (lead V_5) 0.08 sec; positive delta wave all chest leads

LOWN-GANONG-LEVINE

Lown-Ganong-Levine (LGL)

CRITERIA

- Short PR interval (due to James fiber from atrium into His bundle which bypasses AV node delay)
- No delta wave (normal QRS complex)

CLINICAL SITUATIONS

- Congenital

Note. Lown-Ganong-Levine predisposes to supraventricular tachycardia

DIFFERENTIAL DIAGNOSIS

- Wolff-Parkinson-White
- Premature atrial contraction
- Low atrial rhythm

TREATMENT

None unless associated with supraventricular tachycardia
(see treatment for supraventricular tachycardia)

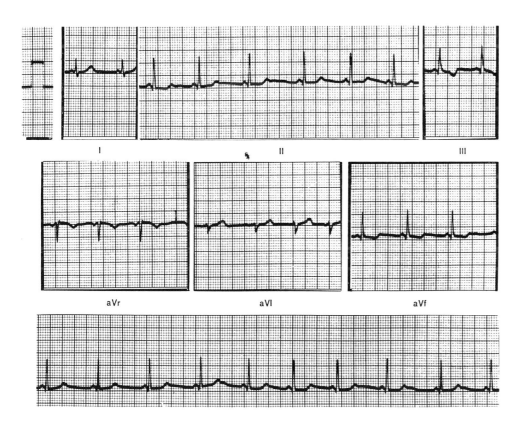

I II III

aVr aVl aVf

Figure 94.

History: 9-year-old girl with infrequent episodes of supraventricular tachycardia; treatment with digoxin reduced the number of episodes.

Interpretation: PR interval (lead I) 0.08 sec; no delta wave

187

Artificial Pacemakers

Atrial Demand Pacemakers

CHARACTERISTICS

Normal pacemaker function

- R-R interval is regular
- QRS rate is set by manufacturer or may be programmed
- When the pacemaker is operational, the pacemaker rate should vary from set rate less than the amount indicated by the manufacturer (see pacemaker manual)
- Most pacemakers operate in a "demand" mode; if the P wave is not sensed at an appropriate interval, the pacemaker will introduce a "spike"
- QRS duration is normal for the patient
- Each paced QRS is preceded by a pacemaker spike and P wave
- Pacemaker spike is narrow (< 0.04 sec) and may obscure the P wave which is caused by the spike
- Spike-to-QRS interval may exceed normal PR interval for the child's age

Abnormal pacemaker function

- Pacemaker failure (battery or generator failure, lead fracture, loss of electrode contact)
  - Return to basic rhythm
  - No pacemaker spikes
- Sensing failure (mechanical failure or deterioration of patient, eg, acidosis)
  - Constant or intermittent, inappropriately timed pacemaker spikes
- Capture failure
  - Pacemaker spikes at an appropriate interval without a following P wave
- Impending battery depletion
  - Pacemaker rate varies from set rate by more than the amount indicated by the manufacturer

INDICATIONS

Note. AV conduction should be proven normal by an intracardiac electrophysiologic study before implantation of an atrial pacemaker.

- Symptomatic: sinus bradycardia, sinus arrest, sino-atrial block
- Overdrive pacing of supraventricular tachycardia or ventricular tachycardia
- Induction of premature atrial contractions to treat supraventricular tachycardia or ventricular tachycardia
- Maintenance of adequate heart rate when medication for tachydysrhythmia causes symptomatic sinus slowing

Figure 95.

History: 8-year-old boy with recurrent supraventricular tachycardia. A pacemaker was implanted because treatment for tachycardia with digitalis, propranolol, and quinidine resulted in sinus bradycardia.

Interpretation: Pacemaker rate 70/min; normal pacemaker function; each QRS complex (QRS) is preceded by a pacemaker spike (Pa) and a P wave (P).

Additional diagnosis: First degree AV block, wide QRS without CRBBB or CLBBB pattern (due to medication)

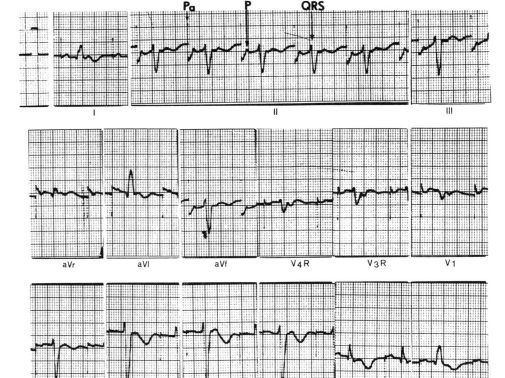

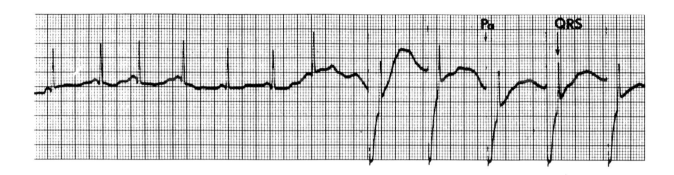

LEAD II

Figure 96.

History:

16-year-old girl, twelve years after repair of secundum atrial septal defect, with a history of atrial flutter; pacemaker was inserted as part of treatment for tachycardia-bradycardia ("sick-sinus") syndrome; pacemaker was set in a demand mode at a rate of 72/min.

Interpretation:

Patient is in an immediate post-exercise recovery period. At the beginning of the tracing, sinus rate > 72/min and the pacemaker is inhibited; with a pause of 0.88 sec (equivalent to a rate of 68/min), the pacer correctly operates in demand mode and begins to introduce spikes (Pa) at rate of 72/min; spike-to-QRS interval is 0.16 sec.

Note. QRS is identical with and without pacing; P waves are not seen because pacing spike is so large.

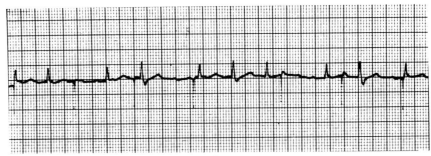

I

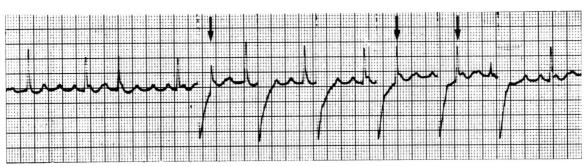

II

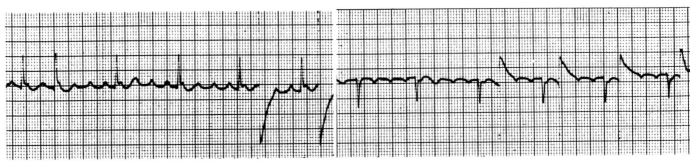

II   AVR

Figure 97.

History: 16-year-old girl—same patient shown in Figure 96

Interpretation: Malfunctioning atrial pacemaker; basic rhythm is atrial flutter; pacemaker fails to sense most flutter waves and introduces spikes intermittently; some of the spikes capture (short R-R intervals following pacemaker spikes) and cause QRS complexes (arrows).

Ventricular Demand Pacemakers

CHARACTERISTICS

Normal operation

- R-R interval is regular
- QRS rate is set by manufacturer or may be programmed
- When pacemaker is operational, pacemaker rate should vary from set rate less than the amount indicated by manufacturer (see pacemaker manual)
- Most pacemakers operate in the "demand" mode; if QRS is not sensed at an appropriate interval, pacemaker will introduce a spike
- QRS duration is prolonged for the child's age (see Table 1)
- QRS morphology: right bundle branch block pattern, usually left ventricular pacemaker; left bundle branch block pattern, usually right ventricular pacemaker
- Each paced QRS is directly preceded by a pacemaker spike

Abnormal operation

- Pacemaker failure (battery or generator failure, lead fracture, loss of electrode contact)
    - Return to basic rhythm
    - No pacemaker spikes
- Sensing failure (mechanical failure or deterioration of patient, eg, acidosis)
    - Constant or intermittent, inappropriately timed pacemaker spikes
- Capture failure (mechanical failure or deterioration of patient)
    - Pacemaker spikes at an appropriate interval without a following QRS
- Impending battery depletion
    - Pacemaker rate varies from set rate by more than the amount indicated by the manufacturer

INDICATIONS REQUIRING VENTRICULAR PACEMAKER
IN SPECIAL CIRCUMSTANCES

Note.   If AV conduction is either abnormal or cannot be proven to be normal by intracardiac electrophysiologic study, a ventricular pacemaker should be implanted for the following indications:

- Symptomatic: sinus bradycardia, sinus arrest, sino-atrial block
- Maintenance of adequate heart rate when medication for tachydysrhythmia causes symptomatic sinus slowing
- Overdrive pacing of supraventricular tachycardia or ventricular tachycardia

INDICATIONS ALWAYS REQUIRING VENTRICULAR
PACEMAKER

- Symptomatic advanced second degree AV block or third degree AV block
- Induction of premature ventricular contractions to treat supraventricular tachycardia or ventricular tachycardia

Figure 98.

History: A 3-month-old boy with a history of congenital complete AV block and a slow ventricular rate with signs of congestive heart failure had a pacemaker implanted at 1 month of age.

Interpretation: Normal pacemaker function; pacemaker spike (Pa) immediately precedes each QRS complex; QRS duration prolonged for age (0.10 sec) with left bundle branch block pattern

Additional diagnosis: Third degree AV block with independent atrial rate 140/min (P); no ventriculo-atrial conduction

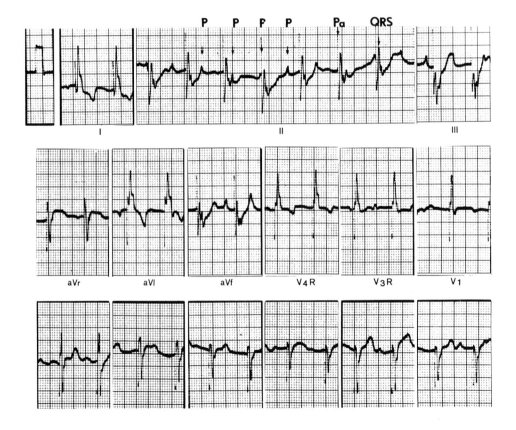

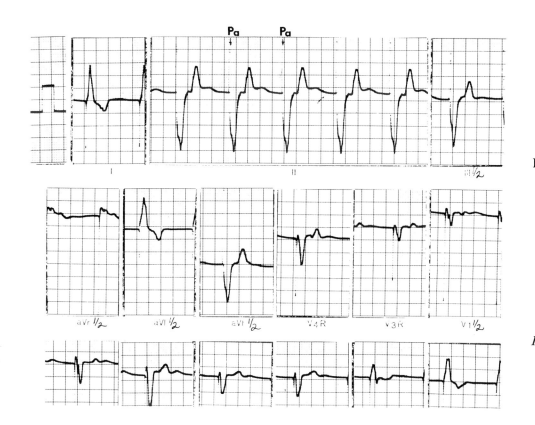

Figure 99.

History: A 9-year-old girl developed tachycardia-bradycardia syndrome one year following repair of ostium primum atrial septal defect. Medication caused extreme sinus bradycardia and a pacemaker was inserted; cardiac catheterization revealed poor AV node function and therefore a ventricular pacemaker was inserted instead of an atrial pacemaker.

Interpretation: Normal pacemaker function; pacemaker spike (Pa) immediately precedes each QRS complex; QRS duration prolonged for age (0.13 sec) with left bundle branch block pattern

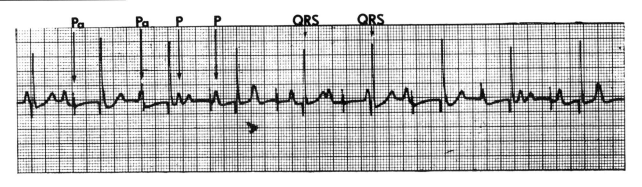

Figure 100.

LEAD II

History: A 3-year-old with double outlet right ventricle and congenital complete AV block had a permanent-demand ventricular pacemaker implanted. He fell off a horse and was found to have a slow pulse rate. The pacemaker was programmed to 65 beats/min to test the programming circuit. At reoperation, the lead had become separated from the heart.

Interpretation: The basic rhythm is complete AV block with the ventricular (QRS-QRS) rate 60/min, atrial rate (P-P) 112/min, and pacemaker rate (Pa-Pa) 65/min. The pacemaker is neither sensing (all Pa spikes should be inhibited) nor capturing (all the abnormal Pa spikes occur at a time when they should capture).

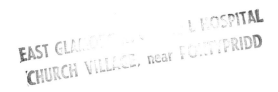